PUBLIC HEALTH IN CHINA SERIES
Series Editor **Liming Li**

Tropical Diseases in China

Neglected Tropical Diseases and Malaria

Editor Xiao-nong Zhou

People's Medical Publishing House

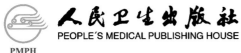

人民卫生出版社
PEOPLE'S MEDICAL PUBLISHING HOUSE

PMPH

Website: http://www.pmph.com/

Book Title: Tropical Diseases in China: Neglected Tropical Diseases and Malaria
(Public Health in China Series)
中国公共卫生：热带病防治实践．被忽视热带病与疟疾（英文版）

Contact address: No. 19, Pan Jia Yuan Nan Li, Chaoyang District, Beijing 100021, P.R. China, phone/fax: 8610 5978 7584, E-mail: pmph@pmph.com

First published: 2019
ISBN: 978-7-117-28427-1

Cataloguing in Publication Data:
A catalogue record for this book is available from the
CIP-Database China.

ISBN 978-7-117-28427-1

Printed in The People's Republic of China

Contributors

Lin Ai
National Institute of Parasitic Diseases
Chinese Center for Disease Control and Prevention
Shanghai, China

Jun-hu Chen
National Institute of Parasitic Diseases
Chinese Center for Disease Control and Prevention
Shanghai, China

Zhi-bin Cheng
Peking Union Medical College
Beijing, China

Li-ping Duan
National Institute of Parasitic Diseases
Chinese Center for Disease Control and Prevention
Shanghai, China

Jun Feng
National Institute of Parasitic Diseases
Chinese Center for Disease Control and Prevention
Shanghai, China

Le-le Huo
National Institute of Parasitic Diseases
Chinese Center for Disease Control and Prevention
Shanghai, China

Bin Jiang

National Institute of Parasitic Diseases

Chinese Center for Disease Control and Prevention

Shanghai, China

Viktoria Khroundina

The Journal *Infectious Diseases of Poverty*

Melbourne, Australia

Kassegne Kokouvi

National Institute of Parasitic Diseases

Chinese Center for Disease Control and Prevention

Shanghai, China

Mei Li

National Institute of Parasitic Diseases

Chinese Center for Disease Control and Prevention

Shanghai, China

Cong-shan Liu

National Institute of Parasitic Diseases

Chinese Center for Disease Control and Prevention

Shanghai, China

Fei Luo

Chongqing Center for Disease Control and Prevention

Chongqing, China

Duo-quan Wang

National Institute of Parasitic Diseases

Chinese Center for Disease Control and Prevention

Shanghai, China

Ru-bo Wang

National Institute of Parasitic Diseases

Chinese Center for Disease Control and Prevention

Shanghai, China

Wei-si Wang

National Institute of Parasitic Diseases

Chinese Center for Disease Control and Prevention

Shanghai, China

Yu-fen Wei

National Institute of Parasitic Diseases

Chinese Center for Disease Control and Prevention

Shanghai, China

Zhi-gui Xia

National Institute of Parasitic Diseases

Chinese Center for Disease Control and Prevention

Shanghai, China

Ning Xiao

National Institute of Parasitic Diseases

Chinese Center for Disease Control and Prevention

Shanghai, China

Guo-jing Yang

Swiss Tropical and Public Health Institute, University of Basel

Basel, Switzerland

Kun Yang

Jiangsu Institute of Parasitic Diseses

Wuxi, Jiangsu, China

Pin Yang

National Institute of Parasitic Diseases

Chinese Center for Disease Control and Prevention

Shanghai, China

Hao-bing Zhang

National Institute of Parasitic Diseases

Chinese Center for Disease Control and Prevention

Shanghai, China

Qi Zheng

National Institute of Parasitic Diseases

Chinese Center for Disease Control and Prevention

Shanghai, China

Zhi Zheng

Peking Union Medical College

Beijing, China

Xiao-nong Zhou

National Institute of Parasitic Diseases

Chinese Center for Disease Control and Prevention

Shanghai, China

Preface

Tropical diseases are prevalent in or unique to tropical and subtropical regions. Some of these diseases are transmitted by insects, some are transmitted through food, or water which makes more poor people to be infected with pathogens. The pathogens in tropical and subtropical climates, including parasite, bacterium, or virus, etc., are infectious sources to humans and animals, through vectors or intermediate hosts in the environment suitable for the development of those pathogens.

The most important tropical disease affecting millions of people is malaria, which is a typical mosquito-borne disease. Neglected tropical diseases (NTDs), meanwhile, are a diverse group of tropical infections that are especially common in the low- and middle-income people in developing regions of Africa, Asia, and the Americas. A total of 20 kinds of diseases defined by the World Health Organization (WHO) in 2017 were listed in the NTD portfolio, including Buruli ulcer, Chagas disease, dengue and chikungunya, dracunculiasis (guinea-worm disease), echinoc-occosis, foodborne trematodiases, human African trypanosomiasis (sleeping sick-ness), leishmaniasis, leprosy (Hansen's disease), lymphatic filariasis, mycetoma, chromoblastomycosis and other deep mycoses, onchocerciasis (river blindness), rabies, scabies and other ectoparasitoses, schistosomiasis, soil-transmitted helmin-thiases, snakebite envenoming, taeniasis/cysticercosis, trachoma, and yaws (endemic treponematoses). Currently, both NTDs and malaria have been listed in the targeted infectious diseases to be controlled in the UN sustainable development goals by 2030, in spite of NTDs are still under attention with limited resources for control activities in developing world, contrasted with the big three diseases (HIV/AIDS, tuberculosis, and malaria) that have generally been received greater funding for treatment and research.

Both NTDs and malaria have never been neglected in China, with significant attention paid, in terms of control efforts, by the Chinese government. For example, in order to clearly map disease transmission patterns and geographical distribution to provide information for decision-makers, the Chinese government has carried out three nationwide surveys on important human parasitic diseases in mainland China. The results of these surveys provided baseline data for the formulation of national NTDs control programs at different periods of time. The first investigation was carried out in 1988–1992, coordinated by the Ministry of Health in order to achieve the "health for all 2000" strategic objectives. The second survey was undertaken in 2001–2004 in 31 provinces, autonomous regions, and municipalities, and had the following outcomes: (i) gaining an understanding of the epidemic status and endemicity of important human parasitic diseases in mainland China; (ii) assessing the burden of human parasitic diseases; (iii) and discovering three new species of human parasites in the country. The third survey in 2014–2016 led to a significant decline in human infections for various parasitic diseases, in line with steps taken in economic development, providing baseline data to achieve the "Healthy China 2030".

The effort in national tropical disease control programme has been integrated with other local development projects and contributed significantly to local economic development. This multi-sectoral cooperation approach to control tropical diseases in China is a typical solution to control infectious diseases undertaken in the developing countries, due to its cost-effectiveness with a lower input and a higher output.

This book is a collection of lessons learnt from the national malaria control program as well as national NTDs control program, which designed to focus on epidemiology, diagnosis and drug development, and well as control strategies of those NTDs and malaria. We believe all the knowledge acquired, technologies used, and policies developed in the national diseases control programs of China are invaluable in terms of its working mechanism. It is expected that, under the concept of "we share common features in society's development" proposed by the Chinese government, the experiences gained through the national disease control programme as well as collaborative researches are easily to be transferred and tailored to the local communities in other low- and middle-income countries.

Xiao-nong Zhou

Contents

Chapter 1

Neglected Tropical Diseases in China

**Li-ping Duan, Qi Zheng, Hao-bing Zhang, Yu-fen Wei,
Lin Ai, Le-le Huo, Wei-si Wang, Hao-bing Zhang,
Cong-shan Liu, and Lin Ai**

1.1 Soil-transmitted helminthiasis

Soil-transmitted helminths are important pathogenic parasites, including ascaris (*Ascaris lumbricoides*), trichuris (*Trichuris trichiura*), and hookworm (*Ancylostoma duodenale* and *Necator americanus*). In China, environmental conditions are suitable for the survival of soil-transmitted helminths, exposing the local population to infection.

With the development of social economy and the improvement of people's living standard, people's diets in terms of a variety of food being available are changing which altered the way to eat more raw food. These allowed for some changes in the prevalence of helminth infections. Based on the Second nationwide survey conducted in 2004, the infection rate of soil-transmitted helminthiasis (STH) was 19.56% in China, comprising 6.12% hookworm infection, 12.72% ascaris infection, and 4.63% trichuris infection. The number of STH infected individuals in China was approximately 129 million; about 39.3 million were hookworm patients, 85.93 million were ascariasis patients, and 29.09 million were trichuriasis patients. Compared with the results from the first national survey conducted in 1990, the standardized infection rates of hookworm, ascariasis, and trichuriasis decreased by 60.7%, 71.28%, and 73.60%, respectively.[1-2] Though achievements have been made, but the large-scale use of insecticides and the universal use of anthelmintic drugs might inevitably lead to a decrease in drug sensitivity, and even to an increase in parasite resistance.

To capture the data on the epidemiology, distribution and epidemic factors of major human parasitic diseases, evaluate the implementation of the National Control Plan for Major Parasitic Diseases (2006–2015), the third nationwide epidemiological survey on parasitic diseases in China was conducted in 2014–2015. The survey covered 31 provinces (autonomous regions/municipalities) (Hongkong, Macao and Taiwan not included) in mainland of China. In rural areas, soil-transmitted helminthiasis (hookworm disease, ascariasis, trichuriasis and enterobiasis), taeniasis, clonorchiasis and intestinal protozoiasis were investigated. Clonorchiasis was also investigated in urban/town areas. A total of 617,441 people were surveyed in 31 provinces of China, in which 484 210 were from rural areas and 133,231 from urban/town areas. The weighted infection rate of major parasitic diseases in rural areas was 5.96%, and the estimated population under infection was 38.59 million, of which 34.3 million were single infection and 4.30 million were mixed infection. The weighted infection rate of helminth was 5.10%, and that of protozoa was 0.99%. The weighted infection rate of STHs was 4.49%, in which hookworm infection was 2.62%, ascariasis 1.36% and trichuriasis 1.02%. The estimated number of infection for hookworm infection, ascariasis and trichuriasis was 16.97 million, 8.82 million and 6.60 million, respectively. The weighted infection rate of *Clonorchis sinensis* was 0.47%, and the population under infection was estimated to be 5.98 million, including 1.52 million from rural areas and 4.46 million from urban areas. The weighted infection rate of *Taenia spp.* was 0.06%, and thus 370 thousand people were estimated to be infected. Of the three macro eco-zones in China, the highest weighted infection rate of STHs was found in the Eastern Monsoon Eco-zone (4.65%), followed by the Alpine and Cold Eco-zone in Qinghai-Tibet (4.15%), and the lowest in the Northwest Arid Eco-zone (0.64%). Among the 46 eco-regions, the highest weighted infection rate was found in Sichuan Basin Eco-region (22.16%), followed by Mountainous Areas in Central Hainan Eco-region (21.92%), and Southwest Sichuan-North Yunnan Eco-region (15.88%). STHs were not detected in the Xiaoxing'an Mountain Eco-region and Sanjiang Plain Eco-region. In 31 provinces of mainland China, the highest weighted infection rate was in Sichuan Province (23.55%), followed by Hainan (12.23%) and Guizhou Province (10.68%).

References

1. Cheng YZ, Xu LS, Chen BJ, et al. Survey on the Current Status of Important Human Parasitic Infections in Fujian Province. Chin J Parasitol Parasit Dis, 2005, 23(5), 283-287.

2. Zhang Q, Li HZ. The Accessibility for Anthelmintic Administration by Different Supply Patterns in Mass Deworming. Chin J Parasitol Parasit Dis, 2010, 28(3), 234-236.

1.1.1   Hookworm

Hookworm infection is one of the three main STH prevalent in China.[1] Hookworm disease is mainly caused by infection with *Necator americanus* or *Ancylostoma duodenale*, and rarely with *A. braziliense* or *Uncinaria stenocephala*. Although effective control strategies have been carried out for 20 years, it still remains an important public health problem in the tropic and subtropic rural areas of China.

Prevalence

In 2006, 576 million cases of hookworm disease were estimated worldwide, of which 39 million were in China.[2] The prevalence of hookworm has fallen down much more rapidly in China, with a reduction rate of 63.7%, much higher than it has worldwide, with a reduction rate of 35.2%, between 1990 and 2004.[3] The Chinese government has devoted a lot of human resources, materials, and financial resources to reduce the prevalence and intensity of hookworm infections in the past 15 years. Since 2006, the prevalence of hookworm in epidemic area were reported decreased by 45.5–92.6%.

In 2015, a third national survey for soil-transmitted helminthiases was implemented in rural China. Totally, 484,210 participants were enrolled in 1,890 sampling units in 604 counties from 31 provinces. Hookworm infections had a weighted prevalence of 2.62% nationally. Hookworm infections were detected in 19 provinces, of which nine exceeded the average. Highest prevalence was found in Sichuan (14.55%) followed by Hainan (8.10%). Overall, 16,974,524 persons were estimated infected with hookworm. Among them, the number of light, moderate and heavy infections was 15,019,422 (88.48%), 952,326 (5.61%) and 1,002,776 (5.91%), respectively. Hookworm diseases were highly prevalent in western and southern China, low endemic in eastern and non-endemic in northern China.

Hookworm infections were highly prevalent in elder, especially those over 60, who had a prevalence over 6%. The prevalence of hookworm infections was 2.29% and 2.96% in males and females, respectively. Out of 3,579 cases with hookworm infection, the cases with single *A. duodenale* infection were 479 (13.38%), the cases with single *N. americanus* were 2,808 (78.46%) and the cases with concurrent infections with both species were 292 (8.16%). *A. duodenale* infection was predominantly endemic in northern areas, while *N. americanus* in southern regions.

Control strategy

In 2005, the Ministry of Health of China issued the "National Control Program on Important Parasitic Diseases from 2006 to 2015", with a target to reduce the prevalence of helminth infections by 70% by 2015. The goals were archived in 2015. A three-pronged approach was proposed to reach this target: (i) undertaking large-scale deworming activities with a benzimidazole; (ii) providing clean water and adequate sanitation; and (iii) implementing health education programs.

Large-scale deworming

The deworming program launched by the Chinese Ministry of Health in 2005 comprises large-scale deworming with effective drugs being carried out in areas where the infection rate of soil-transmitted helminths is more than 50%, with a target population of those aged above three years. Furthermore, chemotherapy is being conducted for selected school-aged children and farmers in areas where the infection rate of soil-transmitted helminths is more than 10% and less than 50%.

In the past 30 years, four kinds of drugs have been used to treat hookworm infections in China, namely levamisole, pyrantel pamoate, mebendazole, and albendazole (Table 1.1).[4, 5] Tribendimidine, a new drug discovered and developed by National Institute of Parasitic Diseases at Chinese Center for Disease Control and Prevention based in Shanghai, has been used in the field recently.

In order to ensure progress in the large-scale deworming program for the control of STH infections (including hookworm), the Ministry of Health selected 12 counties from 11 provinces to conduct a pilot STH control program in 2005.[6] In these pilot areas albendazole or pyrantel pamoate combined with albendazole was

Table 1.1   Drugs used in the regular and periodic treatments of hookworm infections in China.

Drug	Dosage	
	Adults	Children
Albendazole	400 mg once	400 mg once
Mebendazole	100 mg twice a day for 3 days	100 mg twice a day for 3 days
Pyrantel pamoate	20 mg/kg (maximum dose 1 g) for 3 days	20 mg/kg (maximum dose 1 g) for 3 days
Levamisole	2.5 mg/kg once; repeat after 7 days for heavy infections	2.5 mg/kg once; repeat after 7 days for heavy infection
Tribendimidine	400 mg once	200 mg once

administrated twice a year to all residents aged above three years. With 90% compliance rates, the infection rate of hookworm fell by 57% in the program. Taking into account the high rates of post-treatment hookworm reinfections and other factors that limit the success of large-scale chemotherapy programs, it is suggested that large-scale periodic treatment should be conducted in those areas where the rate of STH is more than 50%.[7]

However, even though drug resistance has not yet been clearly demonstrated in human hookworm infections, it is most likely that drug resistance will be introduced if these mass chemotherapy treatment campaigns are sustained. The use of alternative or new drugs are recommended, such as tribendimidine, a new anthelmintic agent registered in China. It was proved that the drug had the similar effect like albendazole when against hookworm in same dosage. Particularly, tribendimidine is more effective against *Necator americanus* while albendazole is more against *Ancylostoma duodenale*.

Sanitation in rural areas

Another objective of the national STH control program is to build hygienic sanitary latrines, with a coverage rate at the county level of above 60% in rural areas by 2010, and above 80% by 2015. This objective was issued based on evidence that the transmission of STH, including hookworm, is extremely difficult to be eliminated in resources limited settings that have inadequate water and poor sanitary conditions, which are exacerbated by a lack of safe water. This goal was finally archived in 2016. In China, many households collect human waste and use it as fertilizer without treating it first. Most people become infected with hookworm while working on contaminated soil. In 1997, about 90% of rural households had latrines, but most were rudimentary and only provided temporary storage of waste. Most of these latrines do not provide any protection from STH infections.

During the past decades, much progress has been made in terms of providing clean water and sanitation. For example, the government has quadrupled investments in water supply and sanitation during the "Five-Year Plan" (2006–2010) period, and latrines have increased markedly in the past two decades (Figure 1.1). In particular, the government has recommended that three-cell latrines be built in rural areas. These are latrines with a three-cell pit, full walls, and a roof in which the pit is airtight and has a cover. Government provided partial subsidy to the family who built the three-cell latrines. Compared with normal latrines, three-cell latrines can reduce morbidity due to helminth infections by about 35% in populations that live in STH endemic areas, by killing 83% of helminth eggs.

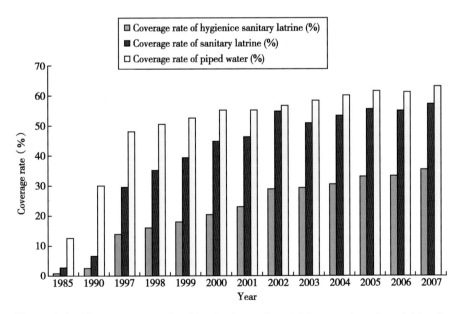

Figure 1.1　The coverage rate of hygienic sanitary latrines and sanitary latrine in rural area of China from 1985 to 2007. (Datas are from the Chinese National Health Commission official website.)

Nine ministries and commissions of the Chinese government have also united to put forward the "Health promotion for farmers" program, with a target to increase the coverage rate of household methane latrines by more than 16% by 2010. This goal was achieved in year 2010. The household methane latrine is one kind of hygienic sanitary latrine that the government subsidizes in transmission areas where helminths are prevalent.[9] It can reduce the concentration of live helminth eggs after treatment with methane more than other hygienic sanitary latrines.[10] Therefore, with the aid of the government, the coverage rate of hygienic sanitary latrines had increased and reached the targets. Building household methane latrines will not only control STH, but will also have important economic benefits. In one year, a methane latrine belonging to one family with four members can provide free heat energy that is equal to 400 kg of standard coal burns, and can also provide seven to ten tons of clean organic fertilizer. All these benefits sum up to US$ 120 per year, which encourages people to reconstruct their latrines as methane latrines.

A marked reduction of hookworm infections was observed after launching this program. In 2002, according to the water and environmental sanitation projects aided by UNICEF, the infection rate of STH in Shucheng County, Anhui Province, was reduced from 28.6% to 17.5% after water supply projects were implemented in the region.[11]

Health education

Another control strategy is giving health education to local residents, with the goal that awareness rate of STH transmission and how to prevent them should be above 70%, and healthy behavior rates should be above 60% and 80% by the end of 2010 and 2015, respectively. This target was drafted because some behaviors, such as working in the field without wearing shoes or eating uncooked vegetables, are directly related to the transmission of hookworm infections. Most people become infected with hookworm because they do not obey hygienic behavior.[12]

In order to reach these targets, local governments made a concerted effort to promote good health-related behaviors. In most rural areas, a network constituted by several non-governmental organizations, such as the National Patriotic Health Campaign Committee, the All-China Women's Federation, and the Communist Youth

League of China, alongside local Centers for Disease Control and Prevention (CDCs) and schools, implemented health education campaigns in order to encourage a wide range of hygienic behaviors.[13] The goal was archived in 2015 by popularizing the knowledge of many basic health behaviors, such as the importance of washing hands with soap before eating and not drinking unboiled water.

Diagnosis

In spite of these developments, there are still dozens of millions of hookworm patients in China, all of them tested by Kato-Katz smears. The Kato-Katz method is a golden standard to test for hookworm infection, but it cannot avoid a certain amount of false-negative results. Therefore, it is very important to develop or introduce new kinds of diagnostic tools for hookworm infection in China. Unfortunately, no approved diagnostic kits by the Chinese Food and Drug Administration (CFDA) were found when querying through the CFDA website (http://www.sfda.gov.cn/WS01/CL0001/).

Various research on diagnostic developments for hookworm infection is currently being conducted. For example, Wang JX and colleagues introduced a quantitative polymerase chain reaction (PCR) method for detecting hookworm infection and for quantification. The real-time PCR method was designed based on the ribosomal DNA intergenic region II of the hookworm *N. americanus*. The detection limit of this method was also compared with the microscopy-based Kato-Katz method.[14]

The real-time PCR method was used to conduct an epidemiological survey on hookworm infection in Fujian, a southern province of China.[6] The real-time PCR method was specific for detecting *N. americanus* infection, and was more sensitive than conventional PCR or a microscopy-based method. A preliminary survey for hookworm infection in villages of Fujian confirmed the high prevalence of hookworm infection in the resident population. In addition, it was found that the infection rate in women was significantly higher than in men.

The real-time PCR method has increased detection sensitivity resulting in more accurate epidemiological studies of hookworm infections, especially when the intensity of the infection needs to be considered.[15] A study was conducted to demonstrate and understand the acquired immunity in golden hamsters (*Mesocricetus aura-tus*) elicited by primary *N. americanus* infective third-stage larvae (L3). Hamsters infected with 150 L3 for one, two, three, six, and ten weeks were challenged with the same number of L3 and sacrificed 25 days post-challenge. The hamsters that were infected initially exhibited 99–100% protection against the subsequent L3 challenge compared to uninfected naïve hamsters. The acquired immunity was developed as early as one week post L3 infection and lasted up to ten weeks. Similar protective immunity was obtained in hamsters infected with *N. americanus* L3 and then treated orally with a single dose of 100 mg/kg albendazole, followed by challenge with *N. americanus* L3 four and eight weeks post-treatment. The infected hamsters exhibited a rise in immunoglobulin (Ig) G antibodies against L3 and juvenile adult worm antigens. A histological examination showed that the challenging L3 were trapped in the skin of initially infected hamsters and surrounded or infiltrated by different inflammatory cells. The trapped L3 were either damaged or dead, followed by the formation of granulomas encasing dead worms. The results demonstrate that hamsters primarily infected with *N. americanus* L3 develop acquired immunity against reinfection.

Chinese scientists explored the possibility of using specific antigens for the immunodiagnosis of hookworm infection in endemic areas. Infective L3 of the canine hookworm, *Ancylostoma caninum*, were prepared as the source of antigen. The enzyme-linked immunoelectrotransfer blot technique has been employed as an immunodiagnostic method. Two immunodominant bands of hookworm antigens (42 kDa and 55 kDa) were recognized by the sera of hookworm-infected patients (serum dilution 1:200; antigen centrifuged at 36,000 r/m for 20 minutes), but not by the sera of negative controls. The 42 kDa and 55 kDa *A. caninum* antigens might be the specific antigens that could be used for the immunodiagnosis of hookworm infection in endemic areas.

Table 1.2 shows the number of publications that were obtained by searching the Chinese databases, China National Knowledge Infrastructure (CNKI, http://www.cnki.net/) and Wanfang (http://www.wanfangdata.com.cn/index.html), using the keywords (hookworm + diagnosis + endemic/survey/site/screening), from January 2008 to January 2017.

Table 1.2　Numbers of the publications mentioning specific keywords obtained by searching the CNKI and Wanfang databases.

Keywords	CNKI	Wanfang
Endemic	27	23
Survey	31	42
Site	10	1
Screening	4	0

Based on the above results, it was found that the following methodologies have been used in epidemiological surveys: (i) endoscope/small bowel capsule endoscopy/gastroscopy; (ii) enzyme-linked immunosorbent assay (ELISA); (iii) eggs detection under microscopy; (iv) Kato-Katz method; (v) *in vitro* culture using filter paper for larvae identification; (vi) saturated salt flotation method; (vii) PCR; (viii) antigen test; and (ix) anemia examination as clinical indicators (Table 1.3).

Table 1.3　The diagnostic reagents/methods mentioned in the publications.

Diagnostic reagents/methods	Number
Endoscope/small bowel capsule endoscopy/gastroscopy	3
ELISA	2
Eggs under microscopy	1
Kato-Katz	4
In vitro filter paper method	2
Saturated salt flotation method	4
PCR	2
Antigen skin test	2
Indicators of anemia	1
Total	21

Treatment

The Chinese Ministry of Health issued "Technical protocols of hookworm control and prevention" in 2010 which recommend to use tribendimidine, albendazole, pyrantel and compound albendazole tablets (Table 1.4).

Table 1.4　Recommended drugs and their dosage for the treatment of intestinal hookworm (*Necator americanus* and *Ancylostoma duodenale*) infection in China.

Drugs	Dosage	
	Adults	Children and juvenile
Tribendimidine	≥14 years of age, 400 mg once	3–14 years of age, 200 mg once
Albendazole*	≥12 years of age, 400 mg once	3–12 years of age, 200 mg once
Pyrantel pamoate	≥12 years of age, 1.2–1.5 g once	2–12 years of age, 10 mg/kg once
Compound albendazole*	≥7 years of age, 2 tablets once	2–6 years of age, 1.5 tablets once

*Each tablet of compound albendazole contains 67 mg albendazole and 250 mg pyrantel pamoate.

Note: Pregnant women, nursing mothers and children<2 years of age are not recommended to be treated.

References

1. Montresor A, Cong DT, Sinuon M, et al. Large-scale preventive chemotherapy for the control of helminth infection in Western Pacific countries: six years later. PLoS Negl Trop Dis, 2008, 2: e278.

2. de Silva NR, Brooker S, Hotez PJ, et al. Soil-transmitted helminth infections: updating the global picture. Trends Parasitol 2003, 19: 547-551.

3. Hotez PJ, Bethony J, Bottazzi ME, et al. Hookworm: "the great infection of mankind". Plos Med, 2005, 2: e67.

4. Ge GX, Zhong YP. A case infected with three kinds of soil-transmitted helminths. Zhongguo Ji Sheng Chong Xue Yu Ji Sheng Chong Bing Za Zhi, 2011, 29: 332, 338.

5. Zu LQ, Jiang ZX, Yu SH, et al. Treatment of soil-transmitted helminth infections by anthelmintics in current use. Zhongguo Ji Sheng Chong Xue Yu Ji Sheng Chong Bing Za Zhi, 1992, 10: 95-99. (In Chinese)

6. Chen BJ, Li LS, Zhang RY, et al. Surveillance on the prevalence of soil-transmitted nematode infection in Fujian in 2006-2010. Zhongguo Ji Sheng Chong Xue Yu Ji Sheng Chong Bing Za Zhi, 2012, 30: 52-55. (In Chinese)

7. Quinnell RJ, Slater AF, Tighe P, et al. Reinfection with hookworm after chemotherapy in Papua New Guinea. Parasitology, 1993, 106 (Pt 4): 379-385.

8. Xiao SH, Hui-Ming W, Tanner M, et al. Tribendimidine: a promising, safe and broad-spectrum anthelmintic agent from China. Acta Trop, 2005, 94: 1-14.

9. Zhu T, Jiang T, Chao N, et al. Effect of soil-transmitted helminthes control through mass deworming and latrine improvement. Zhongguo Xue Xi Chong Bing Fang Zhi Za Zhi, 2015,

27: 510-512. (In Chinese)

10. Xu BS, Wang Y, Dong J, et al. Soil-transmitted nematode infections and cognitive behavior in rural residents of Dezhou City in 2011. Zhongguo Xue Xi Chong Bing Fang Zhi Za Zhi, 2014, 26: 314-315, 322. (In Chinese)

11. Li XM, Chen YD, Xu LQ, et al. Study on a new prevention and control model on soil-borne parasitic diseases in rural areas of China. Zhongguo Xue Xi Chong Bing Fang Zhi Za Zhi, 2011, 23: 719-721.

12. Sun DK, Zhang CP, Chen DZ, et al. Evaluation of integrated control measures for soil-transmitted nematodiasis in Jinhu County, Jiangsu Province. Zhongguo Xue Xi Chong Bing Fang Zhi Za Zhi, 2014, 26: 69-71. (In Chinese)

13. Wang XB, Wang GF, Zhang LX, et al. Correlation between soil-transmitted nematode infections and children's growth. Zhongguo Xue Xi Chong Bing Fang Zhi Za Zhi, 2013, 25: 268-274. (In Chinese)

14. Wang JX, Huang JW, Ye X, et al. SYBR Green PCR detection on hookworm. Chinese Journal of Zoonoses, 2010, 12: 1110-1113. (In Chinese)

15. Lan S, Min-Jun H, Zeng-Zhu G. Overview of global epidemiology and control of soil-transmitted helminth infections. Zhongguo Xue Xi Chong Bing Fang Zhi Za Zhi, 2011, 23: 585-589. (In Chinese)

1.1.2 Ascariasis

Ascariasis is the most common parasitic disease caused by infections with *Ascaris lumbricoides* in the small intestine or other organs of the body.[1] Children are easily infected through the consumption of food contaminated by worms' eggs. According to the clinical manifestations of parasitic or invasive sites, the extent of the infection differs greatly; when worms limited to the intestine, we called them as intestinal ascariasis. The majority of intestinal ascariasis infections are without symptoms, while some patients have varying degrees of gastrointestinal symptoms. *Ascaris* worms enter the bile duct, pancreas, appendix, liver, and other organs, or migrate to the lungs, eyes, brain, thyroid, spinal cord, and other organs, possibly causing corresponding atopic lesions. Severe cases can cause cholangitis, pancreatitis, appendicitis, intestinal obstruction, intestinal perforation, peritonitis, and other complications.[2, 3] When *Ascaris* worms infect humans, both the larvae and adult worms can cause disease in the human body. If larvae are in the human body during the entire migration, it can infect the intestinal system, liver, lungs, and microvascular and lymphoid tissue, which can cause mechanical damage.[4] The metabolites of the larvae are antigens to the human body, as such, can cause systemic allergy symptoms when people are infected. In severe infections, larvae can enter the systemic circulation, invade multiple organs, and causes ectopic damage. The main pathogenic stage of enterobiasis is the adult stage. Adults mainly parasitize in the human intestine, thereby seizing nutrients and affecting human digestion and absorption.[5] Their excretions are also susceptible to allergic reactions. Occasionally, large numbers of parasites can cause intestinal obstruction. In addition, if many worms parasitize the biliary, pancreatic duct, or appendix, this can be fatal.

Epidemiology

The prevalence of ascariasis in China has been reported for a long time. As early as 2,400 years ago, traditional medicine books had a record of ascariasis. The books called it "comparative", "long-worm" and "disturbing worm". During the Ming Dynasty, a Chinese traditional medicine book described ascariasis in more detail, saying it can "cause abdominal pain, vomiting saliva foam, resulting in [the patient] eating less and [becoming] thin".

The state successfully conducted three nationwide major parasitic surveys in 1992, 2004, and 2016 respectively. It is estimated that 531 million people were infected with ascariasis in 1992, with up to 190 million of these aged under 14 years.[6] Ascariasis patients or carriers are the main source of infection. Each female worm lays hundreds of thousands of eggs per day. Fertilized eggs cannot be developed in the human intestine, and must be developed in the outside environment as they need a suitable condition characterized by a certain temperature, humidity and air. Animals and insects such as pigs, dogs, chickens, cats, rats, flies, and the like may also be the source of infection as they may carry the eggs after eating the worms, or come into contact with contaminated human excrement. People can be infected in many ways, mainly by swallowing infective *Ascaris* eggs. Manure and stool are the main ways for roundworm to eggs contaminate the soil.[7, 8] Pigs, flies, and contaminated soil can also spread *Ascaris* eggs. Farmland labor or other means of contact with contaminated soil may result in a large number of human infections. Eggs can enter the mouth via the consumption of vegetables with live eggs, for example, melons and the like, or via swallowed dust.[9] Ascariasis directly affects the infected person's nutritional status, endangers the growth and development of young people, and can cause clinical complications. In China, all levels of government and health departments are increasingly involved in ascariasis control and prevention.[10]

In 1994, there is a widespread distribution of ascariasis in China: from south to north; vertical across the tropical and subtropical, warm temperate, temperate, and boreal areas; and the Qinghai-Tibet Plateau special temperature zone. Infection rates in 1994 were highest in the tropics, followed by the subtropics, warm temperate, temperate, boreal, and the Qinghai-Tibet Plateau. In terms of sex distribution, the average infection rates were similar between men and women. In terms of age distribution, the infection rates were the highest among 5–9-year-olds and decreased with increasing age.[11] With regard to the occupation of infected individuals in 1994, students had the highest infection rates, while fishermen had the lowest, peasants, preschool children and pastoralists, and a family aggregation distribution was observed at the same time.

Until the 1990s, the infection rate of ascariasis among rural people in most areas of China was as high as 60–90%. The positive rates of ascariasis in Huishui County, Guizhou Province; Longhua County, Hebei Province; and Minhe County, Qinghai Province were 83.2%, 64.4%, and 70.5%, respectively. The average infection rate in each province ranged from 6.027% to 71.115%. Infection rates in rural areas are higher than in cities, and are higher in children than in adults. Primary and secondary school students in rural areas had infection rates of 13.53–41.36%; in urban areas, this was 4.88–18.73%.

At the end of January 2001, the Ministry of Health (MoH) of China investigated the status of major parasitic diseases in the country in all regions except for Taiwan, Hong Kong, and Macao. For ascariasis, the MoH examine about 343.5 thousand people in 31 provinces and autonomous regions. In year 2004, it was estimated that more than 85.93 million people were infected with ascariasis. Compare to year 1992, the infection population decreased about 83.8%. It was found that the central and western regions were areas of high infection. The highest infection rates were

Guizhou 42.00%, Hunan 30.86%, Sichuan 27.65%, Hubei 26.86%, and Guangxi 23.26%.

In 2015, the third national survey showed that ascariasis had a weighted prevalence of 1.36% nationally. Ascariasis were detected in all 31 provinces, of which nine exceeded the average. Highest prevalence was found in Sichuan (6.83%), followed by Guizhou (6.15%). Overall, 8,826,171 were estimated infected with *A. lumbricoides*. Among them, the number of light, moderate and heavy infections was 6 147,884 (69.66%), 2,100,937 (23.80%) and 577,351 (6.54%), respectively.

Ascariasis were highly prevalent (over 5%) in western regions but low endemic in northern and eastern areas. Ascariasis was highly prevalent in those aged less than 20. The prevalence in 0–4, 5–9, 10–14 and 15–19 was 1.66%, 1.94%, 2.20% and 1.70%, respectively. The prevalence of ascariasis was 1.25% and 1.48% in males and females, respectively.

Control strategy

As humans normally lack any innate specific immunity to parasites, taking the necessary protective measures for susceptible populations is the best way to prevent parasitic infections.[14] The key to prevention lies in the strengthening of health education; changing bad eating habits and behaviors, such as washing hands before meals, drinking boiled water, and washing fruits and vegetables; and raising people's awareness of self-protection. On the one hand, educating kindergarten- and school-aged children is ideal for starting health education as large numbers can be reached collectively. On the other hand, adolescence is the best time for personal habits to be developed and training to be conducted in order to strengthen health education.

Another prevention and control method is strengthening the monitoring of the epidemic situation of soil-transmitted, including monitoring population incidence, the rectors, intermediate host, and animal hosts helminthes and migrant population, especially for floating populations. If a rise in soil-transmitted helminth disease is found, measures should immediately be taken to control their spread and prevalence. In endemic areas, specific prevention and treatment programs should also be formulated on the basis of the prevalence of the disease: the focus should be on strengthening the management and protection of water sources and paying attention to food hygiene and changing bad eating habits. Prevention and control measures also include the construction of pollution-free toilets to carry out health education. The prevalence of ascariasis has three basic links to the transmission of disease, including infection source, transmission route, and susceptible population. The basic principle of prevention and control is to block these three links. In theory, if you cut off any one link, you can stop the epidemic of disease, but due to the widespread prevalence of ascariasis, there are currently no any measure in place to break the cycle. Therefore, comprehensive prevention and control measures must be considered in terms of controlling the source of infection, cutting off the transmission, and protecting susceptible populations organically in order to effectively control and eliminate ascariasis.[15]

Since important parasitic diseases in China have begun to be investigated, the outcomes of prevention and control of soil-transmitted helminthes in various places have been very impressive. Many localities have accumulated a great deal of experience in terms of controlling the sources of infection and treating patients and those infected.

The source of infection is the main link in the spread of parasitic diseases. In endemic areas, censuses are used to identify the infected people and treat patients. For the people who are in close contact with infected patients, deworming drugs should also be given to avoid contact with the infection, and to control or eliminate the source of infection. By strengthening the management of latrines and water, and paying attention to the environment and personal hygiene, the route of transmission of soil-transmitted helminthes can be broken. In mountainous and rural areas, water supply and toilet building projects are vigorously carried out. Measures that keep drinking water sources clean and not polluted are well worth for the country's investment. Susceptible people should be protected. Some intervention measures and experiences are outlined below:

- Albendazole is not recommended to use for infants and young children below two years old. Also, staple food of children less than 2 years old are normally milk, because the staple food is relatively clean and simple, so most of the parents are ignored to examine the infection condition of their children at this stage. However, the infection rate in infants with ascariasis can be higher than that of the general population, and the number of eggs per gram of pest increases with age. From the perspective of hygiene habits and self-control ability, infants and young children also contribute to environmental soil pollution and have a high chance of being repeatedly infected. Therefore, infants and young children should be regarded as an important source of infection for ascariasis.[16]

- A repeated trail of chemotherapy in one area in China normally lasts for three to ten years. Thus, in a spring and autumn trial during successive years of repeated trials of chemotherapy, in addition to the observed significant reduction in the rate of ascariasis infection, the rate of unfertilized *Ascaris* eggs was increased at the same time. As chemotherapeutic drugs are more sensitive in males, this may also affect the reproductive process of parasites. However, the practical significance of this phenomenon is that chemotherapy can play an important role in controlling the transmission of ascariasis by directly or indirectly reducing the threat of infection.[17]

- *Ascaris*, as one of soil-transmitted helmithes, are contaminated by roundworm eggs in indoor and outdoor environments, which become one of the important factors for the transmission of ascariasis. The infection rate of ascaris in the community is highly positively correlated with the positive rate of *Ascaris* eggs in soil both in and outside the community. Longitudinal observation in the year 2010 confirmed that repeated chemotherapy can not only effectively reduce the rate of ascaris infection in the population, but also significantly reduce the pollution of *Ascaris* eggs in soil. Therefore, monitoring *Ascaris* eggs in the soil can be used as one of the indicators for understanding the prevalence of ascariasis, and the effectiveness of its prevention and treatment.[18]

Diagnosis

At present, the Kato-Katz method and the saturated saline flooding method are widely used in the prevention and treatment of ascariasis in various parts of China. The large proportion of unfertilized eggs is not easy to be floated, thus affecting the detection results of this method. Therefore, the detection rate of Kato-Katz method is higher. However, when the infection is still in the stage of larvae translocation, with the parasitism of the single-sex male, or due to the low infection rate in population after repeated chemotherapy, the immunological test can provide effective diagnostic clues. In animal experiments in year 2010, the positive rate of *Ascaris* antibody was about 90% using the enzyme-labeled antigen convection immunoassay in guinea pig serum infected with *A. suum* for two weeks, and the positive rate was about 95%. As such, the result of immunoassay can be very close to the actual infection situation. However, there is 25% cross-reaction between this method and other gut-nematode infections. If further purification of the antigen used is done and the specificity of the method is improved, immunological diagnostic methods are expected to be useful in epidemiological investigations of ascariasis.[5, 19]

Treatment

Deworming treatment is an important measure to control the source of infection. Deworming can reduce the infection rate and the source of infection, and also improve children's health status. Deworming should be conducted in the fall and winter after the peak infection period, which targeting school-aged children. Due to the possibility of re-infection, it is best to deworm once every 3–4 months. Patients with complications should promptly be sent to the hospital for treatment, and not self-medicate, so as not to delay proper treatment.

The drugs that are recommended by the World Health Organization (WHO) for ascariasis are: albendazole, mebendazole, pyrantel pamoate, and levamisole. The first three are widely used MDA in the control program. Other effective agents include tribendimidine. Pyrantel pamoate is normally used for children aged under two years. Albendazole is not recommended for use during pregnancy and children aged less than two years.[20, 21]

References

1. Dold C, Holland CV. Ascaris and ascariasis. Microbes Infect, 2011, 13(7): 632-637.
2. Krige J, Shaw J. Cholangitis and pancreatitis caused by biliary ascariasis. Clin Gastroenterol Hepatol, 2009, 7(5): A30.
3. Silva MT, Costa VA, Pereira TG, et al. Severity of atopic dermatitis and Ascaris lumbricoides

infection: an evaluation of CCR4+ and CXCR3+ helper T cell frequency. Rev Soc Bras Med Trop, 2012, 45(6): 761-763.

4. Dold C, Cassidy JP, Stafford P, et al. Genetic influence on the kinetics and associated pathology of the early stage (intestinal-hepatic) migration of Ascaris suum in mice. Parasitology, 2010, 137(1): 173-185.

5. de Silva NR, Brooker S, Hotez PJ, et al. Soil-transmitted helminth infections: updating the global picture. Trends Parasitol, 2003, 19(12): 547-551.

6. Chao HJ, Jin L, Xu XZ, et al. Effect of mass chemotherapy in late stage of soil-borne nematodiasis control. Zhongguo Xue Xi Chong Bing Fang Zhi Za Zhi, 2012, 24(5): 585-587. (In Chinese)

7. Ziegelbauer K, Speich B, Mausezahl D, et al. Effect of sanitation on soil-transmitted helminth infection: systematic review and meta-analysis. PLoS Med, 2012, 9(1): e1001162.

8. Freeman MC, Garn JV, Sclar GD, et al. The impact of sanitation on infectious disease and nutritional status: A systematic review and meta-analysis. Int J Hyg Environ Health, 2017, 220(6): 928-949.

9. Gao XH, Zeng XJ, Hong XL, et al. Investigation of infections of soil-transmitted nematodes in Fusheng Village of Poyang Lake area in Jiangxi Province. Zhongguo Xue Xi Chong Bing Fang Zhi Za Zhi, 2013, 25(1): 73-75. (In Chinese)

10. Chen BJ, Li LS, Zhang RY, et al. Surveillance on the prevalence of soil-transmitted nematode infection in Fujian in 2006-2010. Zhongguo Ji Sheng Chong Xue Yu Ji Sheng Chong Bing Za Zhi, 2012, 30(1): 52-55. (In Chinese)

11. Chen XJ, Jiang WC, Cao HJ, et al. Surveillance of soil-transmitted nematodiasis in northern Jiangsu Province from 2006 to 2010. Zhongguo Xue Xi Chong Bing Fang Zhi Za Zhi, 2012, 24(6): 726-727. (In Chinese)

12. Chen HY. Investigation on common human soil-transmitted nematode infections in Quanzhou City in 2012. Zhongguo Xue Xi Chong Bing Fang Zhi Za Zhi, 2014, 26(2): 228-229. (In Chinese)

13. Zhang Q, Chen YD, Xu LQ, et al. Effect of control on infections of soil-transmitted helminthes in demonstration plots of China for 3 years. Zhongguo Xue Xi Chong Bing Fang Zhi Za Zhi, 2011, 23(5): 476-482. (In Chinese)

14. Tian HC, Tang M, Xie H, et al. Evaluation on effectiveness of comprehensive control model for soil-transmitted nematodiasis. Zhongguo Xue Xi Chong Bing Fang Zhi Za Zhi, 2011, 23(5): 518-523. (In Chinese)

15. Chen YD, Zang W. Current situation of soil-transmitted nematodiasis monitoring in China and

working keys in future. Zhongguo Xue Xi Chong Bing Fang Zhi Za Zhi, 2015, 27(2): 111-114. (In Chinese)

16. Wang XB, Zhang LX, Wang GF, et al. Soil-transmitted nematode infection of children and its influencing factors in poverty-stricken areas in two provinces of southwest China. Zhongguo Xue Xi Chong Bing Fang Zhi Za Zhi, 2014, 26(3): 279-283. (In Chinese)

17. Wu WY, Xu GF, Lin CZ, et al. Investigation on current status of infections of soil-borne nematodes in Yunxiao County. Zhongguo Xue Xi Chong Bing Fang Zhi Za Zhi, 2013, 25(1): 110-111. (In Chinese)

18. Hui X. Effects of health education on integrated control of soil-transmitted nematodes. Zhongguo Xue Xi Chong Bing Fang Zhi Za Zhi, 2011, 23(5): 595-597. (In Chinese)

19. Li XM, Chen YD, Xu LQ, et al. Study on a new prevention and control model on soil-borne parasitic diseases in rural areas of China. Zhongguo Xue Xi Chong Bing Fang Zhi Za Zhi, 2011, 23(6): 719-721. (In Chinese)

20. Zu LQ, Jiang ZX, Yu SH, et al. Treatment of soil-transmitted helminth infections by anthelmintics in current use. Zhongguo Ji Sheng Chong Xue Yu Ji Sheng Chong Bing Za Zhi, 1992, 10(2): 95-99. (In Chinese)

21. Yang WP, Shao JO, Chen YJ. Effect of chemotherapeutic regimens on soil-transmitted nematode infections in areas with low endemicity. Zhongguo Ji Sheng Chong Xue Yu Ji Sheng Chong Bing Za Zhi, 2003, 21(2): 128. (In Chinese)

1.1.3 Trichuriasis

Trichuris trichiura (whipworm) is a common soil-transmitted helminth that parasitizes the human body. It widely distributed in the warm, humid tropical, subtropical, and temperate regions.[1] In China, trichuriasis is distributed nationwide, with a large number of people infected, especially children and adolescents. If infection is light, for example, if there are less than five worms in a human, symptoms are not easy to observe. When a person has a lot of *Trichuris* worms, the patient may experience abdominal pain, diarrhea (could contain blood if the infection is serious), and anemia.[2] Normally, anemia is highly dependent on the amount of adult worms in a patient's body. In extremely severe infections, adult worms can attach to the rectal mucosa, which can sometimes cause chronic dysentery, with abdominal pain and severe tenesmus, and occasionally lead to rectal prolapse.[3]

The life cycle of *Trichuris* spp. is simple, with people the only host for the parasite. If adult parasites are mainly found in the human cecum, there can be severe infection of the colon, rectum, and even the lower ileum and other places. After mating and spawning at the parasitic sites, the eggs are excreted with the host feces and develop into infected eggs in the soil in about three weeks. The infected eggs can be orally ingested with contaminated food or water. Eggs hatch in the small intestine, invade into the local intestinal mucosa, and affect the nutritional status and development of the human host. After about ten days, larvae return to the intestine to migrate to the cecum, then it will grow up to adult worm (development of adult worm). Spawning from the adult worm takes about one to three months. A female lays about 5,000-20,000 eggs daily. The adult worm's life expectancy is three to five years; elderly worms can live up to eight years.[4]

Epidemiology

From 1988 to 1994 the survey on the distribution of human parasites in China showed, for the first time, that the prevalence of trichuriasis in the population was 19.92%.[5] The report also analyzed and discussed the characteristics of population distribution and geographical distribution. In order to understand the current epidemic situation and influencing factors of human parasitic diseases, the preventive measures and effects after the first distribution survey were evaluated to provide the basis for the formulation of future prevention and treatment strategies.[6]

From 2001 to 2004, the Ministry of Health of China led the investigation on the status of parasitic diseases and related natural and social factors in mainland China. The findings in terms of trichuriasis were as follows: The prevalence of trichuriasis was relatively low and the proportion of those with severe infections was relatively high, as the economic situation is closely related to the local conditions of culture, education, health, environment, and lifestyle. People got infection through dirty drinking water (farm water, stream water, pond water, and pool water), and people using organic fertilizer (mostly human decontamination) had higher rates of infection in the population with lower education levels. Children with unhealthier habits such as eating without washing hands, living conditions and ethnic minorities with poor sanitation status, had higher rates of infection, indicating that trichuriasis is affected by various social and economic factors.[7]

The third national survey showed that trichuriasis had a weighted prevalence of 1.02% nationally. Trichuriasis was detected in 28 provinces, of which six exceeded the average. Highest prevalence was found in Sichuan (6.43%), followed by Hainan (4.30%) and Yunnan (4.18%). Overall, 6,602,163 persons were estimated infected with *T. trichiura*. Among them, the number of light, moderate and heavy infections was 5,752,696 (87.13%), 845,876 (12.81%) and 3,592 (0.05%), respectively. Trichuriasis was highly prevalent in western regions, moderately in central areas, but very low in northern areas. Trichuriasis was highly prevalent in those aged 5–19. The prevalence in 5–9, 10–14 and 15–19 was 1.74%, 2.13% and 1.81%, respectively. The prevalence of trichuriasis was 1.06% in males and 0.97% in females.

Control strategy

Due to the positive effect of social factors, the prevalence of trichuriasis in China has decreased significantly from 19.92% a decade ago to the current rate of 4.63%, a reduction of 76.76%. This decline is due to many reasons. For example, the rapid development of education, culture, and public health is driven by the rapid economic development in the entire country, especially in the vast rural areas of western China.[8] The improvement of the environment and the popularization of health education has meant that the masses continue to change their previously poor diets, as well as lifestyle and health habits. Health needs and self-protection awareness have increased, and prevention and control efforts have been carried out in large areas, blocking the spread of the epidemic. As in the first nationwide survey in 1994, the prevalence of trichuriasis in that survey was still found to be higher in women than in men. The age group of 5–15 years had a higher rate of infection than the other age groups. Fishermen were more likely to have the infection as compared to other occupations, and other ethnic minorities were more likely to be infected than those of the Han ethnic group. This may be related to the nature of work that women do, the level of education, the health habits of children and adolescents, the living environment of ethnic minorities, and other lifestyle and eating habits. More attention should be paid to these factors in future, for the prevention and control of trichuriasis.

Although soil-transmitted helmithes are not belong to a notifiable infectious disease which should be reported to the government every month, the Ministry of Health of China, and the Chinese Center for Disease Control and Prevention (China CDC) has listed the soil-transmitted helmithes into the national key communicable diseases and vector bio-monitoring systems in 2006 due to their wide distribution and large number of infections. According to survey results released by the Ministry of Health in 2005, ten monitoring points (of one kind) were set up in highly endemic areas with infection rates of soil-transmitted helmithes >20%: Hainan, Guizhou, Sichuan, Guangxi, Hunan Chongqing, Fujian, Hubei, Jiangxi, and Yunnan. Seven monitoring points (type II monitoring points) were established in moderately endemic areas with an infection rate of 5–20%: Anhui, Guangdong, Shandong, Gansu, Qinghai, and Jiangsu. Five monitoring points were set up (three types of monitoring points) in low endemic areas with infection rates of <5%: Heilongjiang, Shanghai, Hebei, Shanxi, and Beijing.[9]

Some autonomous regions and municipalities took the initiation of the national monitoring work as an opportunity to successively set up provincial-level monitoring sites. Until the end of 2017, more than 300 provincial monitoring sites were established. According to the data of these monitoring sites, the trichuriasis infection rate has dropped from 5.88% in 2006 to 0.42% in 2013, a decrease of 92.86%. The monitoring sites in Yunnan, Guizhou, Jiangxi, Hainan, and Shandong showed a higher rate of trichuriasis. Among the infections, the proportion of severe infections was 0.40% in 2006, with no severe infections reported since 2010.

The population infection rate of soil-transmitted helminthes has declined significantly in China and the proportion of severe infections of various species of insects has also dropped to a relatively low level, however, highly infected areas still exist.[10, 11] The government offer special budget for the contribution of soil-transmitted helminthes monitoring spots, especially in highly endemic areas, such as Guizhou and Hainan.[12] Population characteristics of soil-transmitted helminthes infection also change. In recent years, among the three kind of soil-transmitted helminthes, the performance of hookworm infection was significantly higher than that of ascariasis and trichuriasis. At the same time, different regions monitor different worm infections, for example, Guizhou and Gansu have monitoring sites for ascariasis and trichuriasis, whereas

Hainan, Sichuan, and Guangdong have monitoring sites for hookworm.[13] Although the infection rates of soil-transmitted helminthes decrease with the increase of cleaning toilet coverage in some monitoring sites, the detection rate of *Ascaris* eggs in the soil at monitoring sites in recent years has not shown the same decrease patterns as that is the prevalence of roundworms. This suggests that there is still a risk of transmission of soil-transmitted helminthes in the country.[14]

Diagnosis

Direct saline smear use is a common way to identify eggs in the stool, both in the field and clinically. However, other methods are also used, such as natural precipitation, saturated brine floatation method, and quantitative transparent method. Continuous fecal examination is required for three rounds in order to improve the detection rate.

Treatment

The distribution of trichuriasis is often consistent with that of ascariasis, and trichuriasis infections are often multi-worm infections. Therefore, drugs for treatment or deworming are often selected from more broad-spectrum drugs, such as albendazole, mebendazole, etc.[15, 16] However, some broad-spectrum drugs have different efficacy rates against ascariasis, trichuriasis, and hookworm, thus when the infection rates of different parasites drop to a certain level, much attention should be paid to choosing the proper drug against trichuriasis. Research on and development of a new and effective drug for trichuriasis treatment must also be intensified.[17]

References

1. Wright JE, Werkman M, Dunn JC, et al. Current epidemiological evidence for predisposition to high or low intensity human helminth infection: a systematic review. Parasit Vectors, 2018, 11(1): 65.

2. Bundy DA, Cooper ES. Trichuris and trichuriasis in humans. Adv Parasitol, 1989, 28: 107-173.

3. Qian MB, Xia S, Zhou X N. Soil-transmitted helminths in China. Lancet Infect Dis, 2015, 15(11): 1262-1263.

4. Olivero JJ. Case in point. Trichuriasis. Hosp Pract (Off Ed), 1995, 30(2): 39.

5. Zhou Q, Liu CF, Zhang LX, et al. Research progress in soil-transmitted helminth infection control among children at home and abroad. Zhongguo Xue Xi Chong Bing Fang Zhi Za Zhi,

2015, 27(4): 431-435. (In Chinese)

6. Chen YD, Zang W. Current situation of soil-transmitted nematodiasis monitoring in China and working keys in future. Zhongguo Xue Xi Chong Bing Fang Zhi Za Zhi, 2015, 27(2): 111-114. (In Chinese)

7. Xia A, Tao HY, Zhao YM, et al. Effect of comprehensive prevention and control of soil-transmitted nematodiasis in Runzhou District of Zhenjiang City. Zhongguo Xue Xi Chong Bing Fang Zhi Za Zhi, 2014, 26(6): 665-668. (In Chinese)

8. Li LS, Chen BJ, Zhang RY, et al. Prevalent trend of the infection of soil-transmitted nematodes in Fujian Province. Zhongguo Ji Sheng Chong Xue Yu Ji Sheng Chong Bing Za Zhi, 2012, 30(2): 95-99. (In Chinese)

9. Zhu T, Jiang T, Chao N, et al. Effect of soil-transmitted helminthes control through mass deworming and latrine improvement. Zhongguo Xue Xi Chong Bing Fang Zhi Za Zhi, 2015, 27(5): 510-512. (In Chinese)

10. Sun DK, Zhang CP, Chen DZ, et al. Evaluation of integrated control measures for soil-transmitted nematodiasis in Jinhu County, Jiangsu Province. Zhongguo Xue Xi Chong Bing Fang Zhi Za Zhi, 2014, 26(1): 69-71. (In Chinese)

11. Sun RG. Surveillance of soil-transmitted nematodiasis in Xinghua City from 2007 to 2011. Zhongguo Xue Xi Chong Bing Fang Zhi Za Zhi, 2012, 24(6): 733-734. (In Chinese)

12. Lin SX, Wang SQ, Hu XM, et al. Epidemiology of soil-transmitted nematode infections in central mountain area of Hainan province. Zhongguo Ji Sheng Chong Xue Yu Ji Sheng Chong Bing Za Zhi, 2010, 28(2): 160-161. (In Chinese)

13. Tian HC, Tang M, Xie H, et al. Evaluation on effectiveness of comprehensive control model for soil-transmitted nematodiasis. Zhongguo Xue Xi Chong Bing Fang Zhi Za Zhi, 2011, 23(5): 518-523. (In Chinese)

14. Wu WY, Xu GF, Lin CZ, et al. Investigation on current status of infections of soil-borne nematodes in Yunxiao County. Zhongguo Xue Xi Chong Bing Fang Zhi Za Zhi, 2013, 25(1): 110-111. (In Chinese)

15. Yang WP, Shao JO, Chen YJ. Effect of chemotherapeutic regimens on soil-transmitted nematode infections in areas with low endemicity. Zhongguo Ji Sheng Chong Xue Yu Ji Sheng Chong Bing Za Zhi, 2003, 21(2): 128. (In Chinese)

16. Chao HJ, Jin XL, Xu XZ, et al. Effect of mass chemotherapy in late stage of soil-borne nematodiasis control. Zhongguo Xue Xi Chong Bing Fang Zhi Za Zhi, 2012, 24(5): 585-587. (In Chinese)

17. Zu LQ, Jiang ZX, Yu SH, et al. Treatment of soil-transmitted helminth infections by anthelmintics in current use. Zhongguo Ji Sheng Chong Xue Yu Ji Sheng Chong Bing Za Zhi, 1992, 10(2): 95-99. (In Chinese)

1.2 Food-borne parasitic diseases

Foodborne parasites have been consistently reported in the developing and endemic countries. However, the presence of these parasites in the developed world has increased since the late 1980s. Many factors can be attributed to the rise of outbreaks in parasitic foodborne diseases, such as the increase of international travel and population migration, and the globalization of the food supply which brings about changing food habits (i.e. fresh foods and vegetables being consumed).

The top 10 foodborne parasites with the greatest global impact to human health based on criteria defined by the UN's Food and Agriculture Organization (FAO) and the WHO are: *Taenia solium* (pork tapeworm); *Echinococcus granulosus* (hydatid worm or dog tapeworm); *E. multilocularis* (a type of tapeworm); *Toxoplasma gondii* (protozoa); *Cryptosporidium* spp. (protozoa); *Entamoeba histolytica* (protozoa); *Trichinella spiralis* (pork worm); Opisthorchiidae (family of flatworms); *Ascaris* spp. (small intestinal roundworms); and *Trypanosoma cruzi* (protozoa).[1] All these parasites are distributed in China except for *Trypanosoma* spp.

In China, foodborne parasitic infections show a similar trend in increasing patterns. The second national survey on parasitic diseases (2001-2004) demonstrated that the foodborne parasitic infection rate was rising significantly.[2] The most representative disease is clonorchiasis, which is endemic in extensive areas. According to population projections, there are as many as 12.49 million people infected with *Clonorchis sinensis* in China. Compared with the first national survey in 1990, the standardized infection rate of *C. sinensis* increased by 74.85% in the second survey. In Guangdong, Guangxi, and Jilin, especially, the infection rate increased by 182%, 164%, and 630%, respectively. During the third national survey, the weighted prevalence of clonorchiasis was 0.47% nationally, and 5,975,383 persons were estimated to be infected. In 18 provinces, *C. sinensis* eggs were detected. Highly prevalence was detected in Guangxi (6.68%), Guangdong (1.91%) and

Heilongjiang (1.62%). Overall, clonorchiasis was highly endemic in southern and northern China, but low in other areas. According to the second survey, the infection rate of *Taenia* spp. was 0.3%, an increase of 52.5% as compared with the first survey, and it was estimated that 550,000 people were infected with *Taenia* spp. in China.

The other two important foodborne parasites in China are *Toxoplasma* and *Trichinella* infections. The infection rates for these disease were increased by 45.2% and 69%, respectively, between the first survey and the second survey; the estimated numbers of infected people reached 100 million and 40 million, respectively.

The first case infected with *Angiostrongyliasis cantonensis* in humans in China was confirmed in 1984. With the improvement of living standards and the development of the market economy, logistics have become more and more developed, resulting in delicacies being commonly transported from the south to the north of the country, which has diffused the infection source of *A. cantonensis*. Moreover, people's dietary patterns have changed greatly in recent years. For example, many kinds of snails have become available to eat, such as *Pomacea canaliculata*, which has been bred aquatically. Human infections with *A. cantonensis* are in a rising trend along with the circulation of the snails. Cases have been reported in 10 provinces (autonomous regions, municipalities, and a special administrative region), including Heilongjiang, Liaoning, Beijing, Tianjin, Jiangsu, Zhejiang, Fujian, Guangdong, Yunnan, and Hong Kong, where about 90% of the total cases occurred in China. All this demonstrates that foodborne parasitic diseases have become an important public health problem in China.

References

1. Food and Agriculture Organization of the United Nations / World Health Organization (2014). Multi Criteria Based Ranking for Risk Management of Foodborne Parasites. Report of a Joint FAO/WHO Expert Meeting on Foodborne Parasites, 3–7 September 2012, FAO Headquarters, Rome, Italy.

2. National office of investigation on the status of important human parasitic diseases. A national survey on current status of the important parasitic diseases in human population. Zhongguo Ji Sheng Chong Xue Yu Ji Sheng Chong Bing Za Zhi, 2005. 23(5 Suppl): 332-40.

1.2.1 Clonorchiasis

Clonorchiasis is a disease caused by *Clonorchis sinensis*, it is also known as liver fluke disease. About 35 million people worldwide are infected with *C. sinensis*, around 15 million of which live in China. *Clonorchis sinensis* was classified as a definite carcinogen in 2009.

In 1875, *C. sinensis* eggs were found in the intestine of a corpse from the Western Han Dynasty, in Jiangling County, Hubei Province, which demonstrated that *C. sinensis* has existed for at least two millennia in China.

The life cycle of *C. sinensis* includes sexual and asexual reproduction in different hosts. The first and second intermediate hosts are freshwater snails and fish, respectively, which were found by Harujiro Kobayashi and Masatomo Muto in 1910 and 1918, respectively.

Epidemiology

Clonorchiasis is highly prevalent in East and Southeast Asia, especially in China, northern parts of Vietnam, Korea, and the far eastern part of Russia. The first national survey on parasitic infections in humans (1988–1992) was carried out among 1,477,742 people from 2,848 survey sites in 31 provinces (excluding Taiwan, Hong Kong, and Macao). The prevalence rate of *C. sinensis* was found to be 0.31% and the standard prevalence rate was 0.33%. The prevalence rates in the provinces of Sichuan, Hainan, Jilin, Heilongjiang, Anhui, Guangxi, and Guangdong were all higher than that of the national average rate, with the highest infection rate (1.82%) detected in Guangdong.[1] According to the second national survey carried out between 2001 and 2004, the prevalence of *C. sinensis* has significantly increased compared with that from the first survey such as the prevalence of Guangdong, Guangxi, and Jilin rising by 182%, 164%, and 630%, respectively.[2]

A series of investigations have been carried out in different provinces from 2000 to 2012. Results show that the prevalence rates of clonorchiasis in Guangdong, Guangxi, Hunan, Jilin, Heilongjiang, Liaoning, and Zhejiang Provinces were 8.6%, 9.9%, 34.3%, 18.5%, 12.4%, 3.1% and 2.3%, respectively. Sporadic cases were reported in Jiangsu (0.8%), Shandong (0.1%), Anhui (0.4%), Sichuan (0.1%), and

Chongqing (0.2%). No cases were reported in Shanghai. No data are available for the remaining 20 provinces for the last decade.

In the third national survey carried out from 2014 to 2015, clonorchiasis was surveyed in both rural and urban areas. Totally, 617,441 participants were enrolled from 31 provinces. Among them, 3,466 persons were detected with *C. sinensis*, namely a crude prevalence of 0.56%. The weighted prevalence was 0.47% nationally, and 5,975,383 persons were estimated to be infected. In 18 provinces, *C. sinensis* eggs were detected. Highly prevalence was detected in Guangxi (6.68%), Guangdong (1.91%) and Heilongjiang (1.62%). Overall, clonorchiasis was highly endemic in southern and northern China, but low in other areas. The prevalence of clonorchiasis was low in lower age groups and increased following the increase of age until middle aged population. The prevalence was 0.77% in those aged 50–54, 0.70% in those aged 40–44 and 0.68% in those aged 30–34. The weighted prevalence was 0.60% in males and 0.34% in females.

The prevalence and infection intensity of *C. sinensis* vary with age and sex. In general, the prevalence and intensity the infection in males are usually higher than in females, and are highest among 50–59-year-olds. The culture of eating raw fish has a profound effect on the prevalence and intensity of the infection.

A key factor affecting the transmission of clonorchiasis is the distribution of the first intermediate host snails, the most important of which are: *Parafossarulus striatulus*, *Alocinma longicornis*, *Bithynia fuchsiana*, and *Melanoides tuberculata*. As the second intermediate host harbors metacercariae, more than 100 species of freshwater fish have been implicated in the transmission of *C. sinensis*. Most of these fish belong to the family Cyprinidae. Several species of crayfish can also harbor metacercariae of *C. sinensis*, as the second intermediate host, and thus contribute to the transmission of clonorchiasis. Piscivorous animals, especially dogs and cats, serve as reservoir hosts for *C. sinensis*. Dogs and cats can maintain the life cycle of the parasite in endemic areas without the involvement of people.

Clinical manifestation and pathogenesis

The symptoms of clonorchiasis are related to worm burden. Patients with a low intensity of infection often show only mild symptoms or are asymptomatic, whereas patients with a high intensity of infection often show unspecific symptoms, such as nausea, asthenia, headache, indigestion, vertigo, dizziness, diarrhea, or abdominal discomfort or pain. Chronic infection with *C. sinensis* results in various complications in the liver and biliary systems, mainly cholangitis, cholelithiasis, and cholecystitis. The pathogenesis of *C. sinensis* infection includes several factors, such as mechanical injury of the worms through the mucosa of the bile ducts, mechanical obstruction of the bile ducts, immunopathology caused by inflammation, toxic effects of the worms' excretory-secretory products (ESPs), and secondary bacterial infection. The worms' accumulation and the narrowing bile ducts cause sequential bile stagnation, obstruction, and bile pigment deposition, which may give rise to the formation of bile duct stones with eggs or dead worms.

A favorable environment for a secondary bacterial infection is established after cholestasis, especially for *Escherichia coli*, which might cause cholangitis. *Clonorchis sinensis* infection is associated with cholecystitis, consisting of the infiltration of mast cells and eosinophils fibrosis, and mucosal hyperplasia of the gallbladder wall. Consequently, a poor function of the gallbladder causes precipitation of bilirubinate, calcium carbonate crystals, and mucin on the eggs, which causes stone formation in the gallbladder.

Diagnosis

The detection of eggs in feces is the gold standard for diagnosing *C. sinensis* infection. Etiological diagnostic methods of *C. sinensis* normaly examined under microscope after feces as detect materials prepared in various ways, including the direct plating method, water washing precipitation method, inverted precipitation method, zinc sulfate float method, sodium thiosulfate float method, aldehyde ether centrifugation precipitation method, sodium hydroxide digestion method, etheric ether centrifugal precipitation method, and Kato-Katz method, et al. The most widely used technique is the Kato-Katz method due to its low cost, simplicity, and the ability to quantify infection intensity. But it has low sensitivity, especially for detecting low-intensity infections. Therefore, Kato-Katz thick smears are recommended to enhance sensitivity.

Immunological diagnosis for clonorchiasis is usually used as a supplementary method, including intradermal test, complement fixation (CF) test, ring precipitation, flocculation precipitation, gel diffusion test, latex agglutination (LA) test, charcoal agglutination test, staphylococcal protein A coagglutination test, indirect hemagglutination (IHA), indirect fluorescent antibody test (immunofluorescent assay, IFA), enzyme-linked immunosorbent assay (ELISA), diffusion-in-gel ELISA, immunoenzyme staining (IES), and the dot immunogold filtration assay (DIGFA), et al. Intradermal test has been applied since the 1950s for the diagnosis of clonorchiasis and was widely used before the invention of ELISA in the late 1970s. Using crude antigens in ELISA is not ideal due to its cross-reactivity, however, use of ESPs can improve sensitivity. Application of recombinant antigens increases specificity, but results in decreased sensitivity. In addition, antibody detection with ELISA tests cannot differentiate between past and active infections, especially in patients with a high intensity of infection.

In the past few years, PCR has been widely used due to its high performance in the diagnosis of low-intensity infections. A loop-mediated isothermal amplification (LAMP) technique has been developed to detect *C. sinensis* infection in the intermediate hosts. Studies to diagnose human *C. sinensis* infection with LAMP are warranted due to the method's simplicity.

Imaging diagnosis is used as an assistant method in clinical diagnosis. Intrahepatic bile duct dilatation, gallbladder sludge in sonography, and increased periductal echogenicity are important diagnostic indicators for clonorchiasis. However, the infection intensity will affect the diagnostic accuracy. In addition, some indicators will persist for several years after treatment, which renders differentiation between active and past infections difficult.

Vaccines and treatment

Vaccine candidates against clonorchiasis are in the preclinical phase, with a worm reduction rate of 31.5–67.2%, some of which show promising results in rats. Most proteins in vaccine candidates are part of ESPs or tegumental proteins. Both nucleic acid-based and protein-based vaccines have been tested, with the *Bacillus subtilis* spore-based vaccine offering the key advantage of oral administration.

Due to lack of a vaccine against clonorchiasis and the difficulties of changing human eating behaviors, chemotherapy remains the main method for controlling clonorchiasis. Many drugs, including chloroquine, bithionol, furapromide, hexachlo-rophene, dithiazanine iodide, amoscanate, niclofolan, hexachloroparaxylene (hex-achloroparaxylol), and metronidazole have been tested against clonorchiasis before the advent of praziquantel in the late 1970s. The effectiveness of these drugs was only moderate, and many of them were found to be toxic.

Praziquantel is a broad-spectrum anthelmintic, a heterocyclic pyrazine-isoquino-line organism. It has been widely used in the treatment of schistosomiasis, clonorchi-asis, and cysticercosis. Praziquantel was first reported by scientists in China and South Korea as being able to treat clonorchiasis. At present, praziquantel is the only recommended drug for the treatment of clonorchiasis. The efficacy of the drug depends on the treatment schedule and the infection intensity of the patient. Usu-ally 25 mg/kg of praziquantel is administered thrice daily for one or two consecutive days, which can be highly efficacious. A total dose of 150 mg/kg will result in a cure rate of 90% or more and an almost 100% egg reduction. A treatment schedule of three doses of 25 mg/kg of praziquantel for one day also results in high egg reduc-tion rates. However, cure rates are low, especially in the treatment of patients with heavy infections. Transient and mild adverse events are usually reported, such as headache, abdominal pain, and dizziness. Although praziquantel resistance had not yet been reported, a study found that the cure rate of 29% was achieved during treat-ment with the recommended dose of praziquantel in Vietnam. Therefore, a particular attention should be paid to an eventual drug resistance.

In addition to praziquantel, albendazole and tribendimidine show good thera-peutic effects against *C. sinensis* in many animal experiments and clinical trials. Albendazole is a broad-spectrum anthelmintic drug with low toxicity. In the 1980s, albendalole showed good therapeutic effects on clonorchiasis, with the efficacy and safety confirmed by further clinical trials. A total dose of 2,800 mg for seven days can achieve cure rates of more than 90%.[3] A comparison study showed that alben-dazole and praziquantel can achieve similar efficacy in the treatment of clonorchi-asis with less adverse events. Tribendimidine, discovered by Chinese scientists, was approved by Chinese authorities for treating helminthiasis in 2004. Tribendimidine is effective for treating *C. sinensis* in hamsters and rats. Mean worm burden reductions were 100% and 98%, after single doses of 100 and 150 mg/kg were administered to rats and hamsters, respectively.[4] Tribendimidine also showed effective activity in juvenile *C. sinensis* in hamsters, with a 90.6% worm burden reduction rate at a dose of 100 mg/kg.[5] In clinical trials, tribendimidine also showed good therapeutic effects against *Opisthorchis viverrini*, and only showed mild and transient adverse effects. Recently, Chinese scientists carried out two randomized controlled trials to assess the efficacy and safety of tribendimidine against *C. sinensis*. Tribendimidine achieved cure rates of 44–50% with a dose of 400 mg/kg. Furthermore, if the 400 mg dose is divided into two, the cure rate is still significant at 33%. A three-day regimen of 400 mg tribendimidine administered once daily results in a cure rate of 58%.

References

1. Xu LQ, Yu Y, Xu SH. Distribution and damage of human parasites in China. Beijing: People's Medical Publishing House, 1999. (In Chinese)

2. CONSIHPD (Coordinating Office of the National Survey on the Important Human Parasitic Diseases). A national survey on current status of the important parasitic diseases in human population. Chin J Parasitol Parasitic Dis, 2005, 23(5 suppl): 332-340. (In Chinese)

3. Cao WJ, Zhong HL, Feng ML. The observation of albendazole treatment for clonorchiasis in 50 patients. Chin J Int Med, 1985, 24 (6): 353-354. (In Chinese)

4. Fürst T, Duthaler U, Sripa B, et al. Trematode infections: liver and lung flukes. Infect Dis Clin North Am, 2012, 26(2): 399-419.

5. Xiao SH, Xue J, Xu LL, et al. Comparative effect of mebendazole, albendazole, tribendimi-dine, and praziquantel in treatment of rats infected with *Clonorchis sinensis*. Parasitol Res, 2011, 108: 723-730.

1.2.2　Teniasis and cysticercosis

1.2.2.1　Teniasis

The adult worms of *Taenia* spp., such as *Taenia solium*, *T. saginata*, and the newly discovered *T. asiatica*, are parasites that live in the human intestine, causing serious disease. Pigs, wild boar, sheep, dogs, bears, monkeys, and some other animals are the intermediate hosts of *T. solium*; cattle and buffalo are the intermediate hosts of *T. saginata*; and pigs, calves, and goats are the intermediate hosts of *T. asiatica*. If a human ingests cysticercus carried by pigs, cattle, or other intermediate hosts, he/

she can become infected with *Taenia* spp. In contrast to infections with *T. saginata* and *T. asiatica*, in which the adult worm only parasitizes the human body, humans themselves can become infected with the larval stages or cysticerci of *T. solium* by swallowing eggs found on contaminated food or by self-infection from eggs of an adult worm parasiting in humen's own intestines. In addition to colonizing the striated muscle, cysticercus can also parasitize other important organs, such as the brain, eyes, and heart. Therefore, *T. solium* is more harmful to humans compared to the other two species.

Ova of four species of parasites including *Taenia* spp. were found in a male corpse in the No.168 Han Dynasty tomb, Phoenix hill in Jiangling County, Hubei Province, indicating that the teniasis infection was prevalent in China as early as 167 BC.[1] Based on the shape and color of gravid proglottids, the tapeworms were also called "Bai Chong" or "Cun Bai Chong", which means "white worm" or "inch white worm" in ancient medical books. "Cun" is a unit of length about 2 or 3 centimeters varied from different times in Chinese history. Yuan-fang Chao described *Taenia* spp. as "a inch-long, white, small, narrow shaped worm" in the *Treatise on Causes and Symptoms of Diseases* in Sui Dynasty 610 AD. The *Synopsis of Prescriptions of the Golden Chamber* says that "eating pork and beef with cysticerci will have the chance to infecte with inch white worm", which shows that the ancient medical professionals not only understood tapeworms, but also recognized that the infection is caused by consuming raw or undercooked meat. Moreover, three taenifuge herbs were recorded in *Shen Nong's Herbal Classic*, Shang Dynasty. During the Tang Dynasty, 11 known prescriptions could expel the inch white worm, as reported in *Essential Prescriptions Worth A Thousand Gold*. These included betel nut, pumpkin seed, and pomegranate root. The ancient Chinese people made a great contribution to prevention and control of tapeworm infections.

Epidemiology

At the time of the first national survey of parasitic diseases conducted in China in 1990, teniasis was distributed in 27 provinces and autonomous regions.[2] The infection rate varied from region to region: the highest rate was in Tibet (up to 8.66%), while the lowest was in Shaanxi (0.002%). The highest infection rate was found among semi-farm and semi-pasturing populations (up to 5.525%), while the average national infection rate was much lower (0.18%). The ethnic group of Pumi had the highest infection rate (up to 48.27%), followed by the Tibetan (6.9%) ethnic group.

The second national survey conducted in 2001-2004 showed that the egg-positive rate of *Taenia* spp. was 0.28% and the seroprevalence of cysticercosis was 0.58%.[3] An estimated 550,000 people nationwide were infected with *Taenia* spp. Higher infection rates were found in central and western China. The top five provinces with the highest infection rates were: Tibet (21.08%), Xinjiang (0.74%), Sichuan (0.36%), Qinghai (0.11%), Shaanxi (0.04%), and Shanxi (0.04%). Compared with the 1990 survey, the standardized infection rate of *Taenia* spp. increased by 52.49%. The infection rates increased especially in Sichuan and Tibet, by 92.77% and 97.89%, respectively. Currently, with the wide-scale centralized pig feed, and clean food and drinking water supplied to swine, cysticercosis infection has decreased in most parts of northeast and north China. Additionally, the period of pig aquaculture shortened, thereby the risk of *T. solium* infection is significantly lower than it was in the past in the central and northern regions due to the less consumption of raw pork now, especially in the minority in southwest China. The third national survey in 2015 showed that the weighted infection rate of *Taenia* spp. was 0.06%, and thus 370,000 people were estimated to be infected.

In recent years, a special investigation on *T. asiatica* has been carried out in several endemic areas of western provinces and autonomous regions. The findings showed that the new species survives in the southwest provinces and autonomous regions, especially seriously prevalent in Guizhou and Sichuan provinces. In terms of the classification of pathogenic parasite species, *T. saginata* tapeworms were detected morphologically in Wushi County (Xinjiang Province), Lhasa City (Tibet), Yajiang County (Sichuan Province), Mengla County (Yunnan Province), and Congjiang County (Guizhou Province). However, samples from Jundu City (Guizhou Province), Dali City (Yunnan Province), Lanping County (Yunnan Province), and Rongshui County (Guangxi Province) were identified as *T. asiatica*.

Taenia asiatica was first documented in the late 1960s in Taiwan. Several authors reported on the paradox of observing a high prevalence of *T. saginata*-like tapeworms in the native indigenous population living in mountainous areas of Taiwan, as these populations restrained from beef consumption,[4] and meat tested negative for bovine cysticercosis for some time.[5] Ping-chin Fan, a Taiwanese parasitologist, conducted various studies on Taiwanese *Taenia* from 1982 to 1992. The infection rate was found to be extremely high among local people in Taiwan, with the highest rate of 12% and the lowest below 1%. The first case in mainland China was reported in 1995 in Yunnan Province. The main epidemic factors include fecal contamination of water sources on pasture and poor eating habits. After proglottids are expelled, the environment can become polluted by eggs, with wild animals becoming infected, and a complete life cycle developing.[6] *Taenia asiatica* can become epidemic in regions and countries in which people do not consume or eat very little of beef. According to the report by Fan, in 1997, human infection rate in the rural mountain areas of Taiwan was 11%, the average parasite burden was 1.6 per adult in infected humans.[7] The improvement of diagnostic technology (auxiliary diagnosis methods, such as serological examination, molecular tests, and imaging by CT/MRI) has resulted in an increase in the number of cases. In China, this tapeworm is commonly found in the Southeastern China, such as Yunnan and Guizhou provinces.

Diagnosis

Modified Kato-Katz thick smear and Adhesive cellophane anal swab method (for children aged less than 12 years) were used to examine for *Taenia* spp. eggs in the national survey. The questionnaire method to ask about a person's history of defecating proglottids is a simple and reliable method for diagnosis and investigation. Proglottids found in fecal matter are not only the basis of diagnosis, but also can distinguish the species of *Taenia* spp. according to the morphology of the gravid proglottid.

Taenia worms generally do not lay eggs in the intestine; the eggs are released only when the gravid proglottid is ruptured with creeping, stretching, or drawing back. The egg-positive rate determined by stool examination is generally not high. It is not only difficult to find *Taenia* eggs in the feces, it is also difficult to distinguish the species of *Taenia* according to the eggs found in the feces. Therefore, an epidemiological investigation for crowd infection of *Taenia* spp. may show certain deviations only with stool examinations.

For the *Taenia solium* infections, intestinal teniasis is diagnosed by discovering gravid segments and eggs in the stool, and perianal scrapings by microscopy. The diagnosis comprises the following steps, such as: questioning the patient about his/her history of eating raw or undercooked pork; egg examination in fecal sample; gravid proglottids collected and main lateral arms of the uterus counted; and inspecting the evacuated scolex following medication.

With regard to *Taenia saginata* infections, it is important to ask patients about their history of passing proglottids. Commonly, gravid proglottid passed in feces is the first noticed and taken to a physician for diagnosis. The two main diagnostic methods are egg examination in stool, and recovery of the scolex and gravid proglottid after treatment.[8] Clinical manifestations caused by *T. asiatica* were similar to that of *T. saginata* and the same treatment regimen is given as well.[9]

Control strategy

Preventative chemotherapy (PC) is one of the most important strategy to control taeniasis in humans. Mass drug administration (MDA) occurs when the whole population of a predefined geographical area is treated at regular intervals, irrespective of clinical status. In contrast, targeted chemotherapy treats only specific risk groups at regular intervals, while selective chemotherapy screens patients and subsequently treats according to clinical status.[10, 11]

Meat hygiene is fundamental to the prevention of human infection with *Taenia* spp. from both pork and beef. The methods include stringent inspection and correct processing or cooking. In pigs, no incision into the musculature are required for this test; a visual-only inspection allowed if the food chain information indicates that the pigs were raised in controlled housing conditions, reflecting the low risk of porcine cysticercosis within this region.[12] Currently, the legislation for cattle requires both visual inspection of carcass surfaces (external and internal, including the diaphragm) and incision and examination of various cysticerci predilection sites including the mandible, masseters and heart, as well as palpation of the tongue.[12]

Hygiene measures including the use of well-constructed latrines, correct management of sewerage sludge and wastewater, and best practices in animal husbandry all contribute to preventing the intermediate host becoming infected. Poor hand hygiene, such as not using soap to wash hands after defecation, has been associated with greater risk of exposure to porcine cysticercosis.[13] Education and awareness around personal hygiene practices are important in the control of *T. solium*, as human cysticercosis infections can be prevented through stringent hand hygiene to prevent fecal-oral contamination with the infective eggs.

Treatment

In China, semen arecae and omphalia (dried sclerotia of *Omphalia lapidescens* Schroet), rhizoma dryopteris crassirhizomae, pericarpium granati, pumpkin seeds, and the extract of the radical bud of *Agrimoniae herba* have been used to treat teniasis from very early on. Animal experiments have also shown that agrimophol extracted from agrimony has a significant effect against tapeworm that is even better than clinical drugs such as Yomesan® (niclosamide) and Bitin (dichlorobisphenol).[14]

In addition to the traditional drugs, the synthetic drugs currently used to treat teniasis are niclosamide and praziquantel. Dichlorobisphenol and quinacrine have also been used, but not widely.[15,16]

The use of niclosamide to treat teniasis began in the early 1960s.[17] In the United States, clinical trials of this drug to treat cestodiasis were reported at the beginning of the 1970s.[18] Imitation niclosamide was also synthesized at the beginning of the 1970s in China, and was used to treat cestodiasis and teniasis.[19]

The trade name of niclosamide is called 'Mie Tao Ling' in Chinese, meaning to "kill tapeworm quickly and effectively". The oral dose is 2 g daily for five to seven successive days,[20] which results in a cure rate of more than 90%. The tablets should be crushed or chewed before swallowing and can be taken either once or in two doses with a one-hour interval. For patients with a body weight of 30 kg, the dosage is 1 gram daily and it is 1.5 grams for those with a body weight of 30–50 kg. When niclosamide is used to expel *T. solium*, the dosage described above is lethal to the worm, but not to the eggs. Thus, one to two hours after medication, an appropriate laxative should be administrated before the worm is digested, which not only can remove the undigested dead segments from the intestine, but can also avoid the eggs hatching and thereby causing cysticercosis. Administration of a laxative is also an effective method to determine the species of *Taenia* spp. according to the morphology of cephalomere, and, more importantly, can deter incomplete anthelminthic treatment. Magnesium sulfate is often used as a laxative clinically, however, it has been reported that there is no significant difference between using magnesium sulfate and another laxative.

Niclosamide is considered to be a safe anti-tapeworm drug because it is only absorbed in the intestine and has no effect on cysticercus cellulosae.[21] Therefore, it is suitable to be administered to patients with brain cysticercosis and ocular cysticercosis.

Praziquantel is a broad-spectrum anthelminthic medicine used to treat trematodes and cestodes in humans and animals; it is especially effective against adult worms in a parasitifer.[22] The medication regimen in the treatment of teniasis tends to be an oral dose of 10–30 mg/kg, then catharsis with magnesium sulfate at dose of 0.5 g/kg two hours later, or with 200 ml of mannitol at a concentration of 20%. Mirabilite, a traditional Chinese medicine, is also often used as a laxative.

Since ancient times, there has been an assortment of effective treatment methods for teniasis using traditional Chinese medicine.[23] In classical books on this topic, cestodes (including *Taenia* and *Bothriocephalus*) are called "Bai Chong" (white worm) or "Cun Bai Chong" (inch white worm), with "Cun" denoting a unit of length varied in different dynasties, about 2–3 cm. The morphology of the worm and symptoms of diseases were described in detail in those books, and the source of infection and methods of prevention were also precisely understood.

Some classical medical books such as *Jin Gui Yao Lue* (*Essential Prescriptions from the Golden Chamber*), *Zhu Bing Yuan Hou Lun* (*General Treatise on the Cause and Symptoms of Diseases*), and *Shen Ji Fang Xuan* (*General Collection for Holy Relief*) documented that teniasis is related to eating raw beef, pork, and fish. Due to the long history of knowledge about cestodes in traditional Chinese medicine, there is a rich selection (dozens) of effective herbs recorded. A variety of books including *Ben Jing* (*Herb Classic*), *Ming Yi Bie Lu* (*Supplementary Records of Famous Physicians*), *Bei Ji Qian Jin Yao Fang* (*Essential Prescriptions Worth a Thousand in Gold for Every Emergency*), *Wai Tai Mi Yao Fang* (*Medical Arcane Essentials from the Imperial Library*), and *Ben Cao Gang Mu* (*Compendium of Materia Medica*) recorded many anticestode medicines. The *Langya* (a kind of rosaceae plant); omphalia (dried sclerotium of a fungi of *Tricholomataceae*, *Omphalia lapidescens* Schroet); areca; pomegranate peel; pumpkin seeds; and hawthorn, have all been confirmed to have significant activities against cestodes by recent experiments. Among them, areca, pumpkin, and omphalia are widely used, consisting of dozens of prescriptions, such as "Liao Cun Bai Chong Fang" (prescription for the cure of teniasis) documented in *Qian Jin Yao Fang*; "Wan Ying Wan" (myriad applications pill) documented in *Xiu Zhen Fang* (compact prescription); and a proven recipe, "Qu Tao Tang" (cestode-expelling decoction).

The composition of "Liao Cun Bai Chong Fang" is 50 g of both areca and kernels of semen torreya, and 12 grams of fructus ulmi macrocarpae. The herbs are pestled, then soaked for a few hours in 400 ml of water and decocted to 100 ml. For one dose, the decoction is repeated twice, and then the slag is filtered, and merged with decocta. Patients should take the decocta twice on an empty stomach in the morning after fasting from the previous night.

"Wan Ying Wan" consists 800 g each of areca, omphalia, semen pharbitidis, and Chinese rhubarb; 100 g of radix aucklandiae; 50 g of lignum aquilariae resinatum; 400g of fructus gleditsiae; and 400 g of cortex meliae. Areca, omphalia, semen pharbitidis, Chinese herb rhubarb, radix aucklandiae, and lignum aquilariae resinatum are ground to powder, while fructus gleditsiae and cortex meliae are decocted and condensed to a concentrated solution. The powder and the solution are prepared as pills the size of a mung bean. The dose for an adult is 10–13 g, which is divided into two parts and taken twice with sweet water in the morning after fasting. The dosage for children can be reduced according to their body weight.

The contents of "Qu Tao Tang" are very simple: 60–120 g of fresh pumpkin seeds and 30–60 g of areca. Areca is pestled, soaked a few hours in 400 ml of water, then decocted to 100 ml, filtered, and the dregs of the decoction are discarded. The treatment procedure consists of two steps: firstly, chewing the fresh pumpkin seeds or taking the seeds in powder form, and then drinking the areca decoction two hours later. The worm body will be discharged in diarrhea 4–5 hours later. If there is no diarrhea, 10 g of natrii sulfas exsiccatus should be taken after mixing it with water. If the tapeworm scolex has not been expelled, treatment should be done again half a month later. If the worm body is not completely discharged from the anus, do not pull the worm by hand; warm bath water is advised to be used to discharge the worm body naturally. In recent years, prescriptions similar to "Qu Tao Tang" in clinical applications are most common resulting in a deworming rate of more than 90%.

Using "areca" and "tapeworms" as keywords, more than 3,000 publications were found in the "China National Knowledge Infrastructure" database. In practice, different research groups and doctors have modified the regimen more or less based on the prescription of areca and pumpkin seeds to treat teniasis. For example, "Xiao Cheng Qi Decoction" contains 100 g of *Rheum officinale*, 150 g of *Magnolia officinalis*, and 100 g of *Citrus aurantium*, and a Binlang Chengqi decoction with areca. Over the years, the regimen reported by Lanzhou Feng in 1956 has been more widely applied clinically.[24] It is based on an areca and pumpkin seed combined therapy, with magnesium sulfate used for catharsis, leading to a cure rate of up to 100%. Lanzhou Feng studied pumpkin seeds combined with areca and their pharmacological effects of expelling *Taenia*. He showed that pumpkin seeds mainly paralyze the middle and posterior segment of the worm, while areca plays a role in paralyzing the scolex and immature proglottid. Pumpkin seeds make the posterior segment of the parasite become soft due to paralysis. After the areca decoction is taken, the scolex loses the capability of suction. Then, magnesium sulfate increases the peristalsis of the intestine, thus accelerating the discharge of the paralyzed parasite body.

The effects of areca are different against the different species of *Taenia*. The strongest effect is on *T. solium*, in which case the areca can completely paralyze the worm body, especially the forepart. In terms of *T. saginata* worms, areca can only paralyze the cephalosome and immature proglottid, but cannot completely paralyze the gravid proglottid located in the middle segment. Pumpkin seeds act on the middle and end proglottid of the worm. Thus, pumpkin seeds combined with areca can completely paralyze *T. saginata* worms, which can then be easily expelled.

Comparing the three therapies (niclosamide, praziquantel, and areca-pumpkin seeds), the areca-pumpkin seeds combination therapy can expel the intact body of the *Taenia* worms most successfully, and this may be related to the different modes of action of the three medicines in this combination. Areca makes the tapeworm get flaccid paralysis, so that the body become elongated when touched and not easy to break. The body of the worm discharged by praziquantel is often broken and it is difficult to find the cephalomere, which is not conducive to determining the amount of worms infected and for evaluating the theraputic effect. The rate of worm recovery is 53.0–69.0% when treated with niclosamide and the rate of intact worm recovery is much lower, about 30%.

The adverse reaction rate of the three treatment regimens varies according to different reports. The most important is that when praziquantel is administered to patients with cerebral cysticercosis, it is prone to lead to intracranial hypertension or epilepsy unknowingly, and patients with ocular cysticercosis misusing praziquantel could become blind, which is a contraindication of praziquantel. Niclosamide is only not absorbed in the intestinal tract and has no effect on cysticercus cellulosae, thus it is safe for treating teniasis. Currently, there is no domestic production of niclosamide for human clinical use in China. Therefore, the pumpkin seeds-areca therapy is a safe and effective approach for teniasis treatment, especially in large-scale teniasis and cysticercosis control.

References

1. Wei DX, Yang WY, Huang SQ, et al. Parasitological Studies on the Ancient Corpse of the Western Han Dynasty Unearthed from Tomb No. 168 on Phoenix Hill at Jiang County. Acta Acad Med Wuhan,1980, 9(3): 1-6, 107. (In Chinese)

2. Yu SH, Xu LQ, Jiang ZX, et al. Summary of first survey for human parasite distribution. Chin J Parasitol Parasit Dis, 1994, (Special issue1): 2-7. (In Chinese)

3. Wang LD. Current Situation of important Parasitic Diseases in China. Beijing: People's Medical Publishing House, 2008, 54-57. (In Chinese)

4. Fan PC. Taiwan Taenia and taeniasis. Parasitol Today, 1988, 4: 86-88.

5. Ooi HK, Ho CM, Chung WC. Historical overview of Taenia asiatica in Taiwan. Korean J Parasitol, 2013, 51(1): 31-36.

6. Li YL. Human parasitology (Seventh edition). Beijing: People's Health Publishing House, 2009. (In Chinese)

7. Fan PC. Annual economic loss caused by *Taenia saginata asiatica* taeniasis in East Asia. Parasitol Today, 1997, 13(5): 194-196.

8. Silva CV, Costa-Cruz JM. A glance at Taenia saginata infection, diagnosis, vaccine, biological control and treatment. Infect Disord Drug Targets. 2010, 10(5): 313-321.

9. Ohnishi K, Sakamoto N, Kobayashi K, et al. Therapeutic effect of praziquantel against *Taeniasis asiatica*. Int J Infect Dis, 2013, 17(8): e656-657

10. Okello AL, Thomas LF. Human taeniasis: current insights into prevention and management strategies in endemiccountries. Risk Manag Healthc Policy, 2017, 10: 107-116.

11. Gabrielli AF, Montresor A, Chitsulo L, et al. Preventive chemotherapy in human helminthiasis: theoretical and operational aspects. Trans R Soc Trop Med Hyg, 2011, 105(12): 683-693.

12. WHO, FAO, OIE. WHO/FAO/OIE Guidelines for the Surveillance, Prevention and Control of Taeniosis/Cysticercosis. Paris: OIE (World Organisation for Animal Health), 2005.

13. Alexander A, John KR, Jayaraman T, et al. Economic implications of three strategies for the control of taeniasis. Trop Med Int Health, 2011, 16(11): 1410-1416.

14. Pharmacology laboratory of Shenyang College of pharmacy and Pharmacology laboratory of Institute of Materia Medica of Liaoning province. Study on active ingredients for anti-cestode in Agrimonia pilosa, the effect and mechanism of Agrimophol for anti-cestode. Journal of Shenyang Pharmaceutical College, 1974, (1): 19-35. (In Chinese)

15. Jiaxian people's hospital. Five cases of taeniasis treated with thiochlorodiphenol. Shandong Medical Journal, 1973, 1: 49

16. Liang RF. Introduction for a New Drug in Treatment of Taeniasis- quinacrine. Journal of Middle-rank Medicine, 1953, 7: 8. (In Chinese)

17. Tietze A. Short report on clinical experiences with Bayer 2353 in tapeworm infections in man. Die Medizinische Welt, 1960, 17; 38: 1995-6.

18. Perera DR, Western KA, Schultz MG. Niclosamide treatment of cestodiasis. Clinicial trials in the United States. Am J Trop Med Hyg, 1970, 19(4): 610-2.

19. Sun CX. Discussion and Suggestions on Yomesan for expelling *T. solium*. Inner Mongolia Medical Journal, 1985, 5(4): 259-60. (In Chinese)

20. Xu CB, Cao WQ, Zhang YQ. Clinical observation for the treatment of taeniasis with Yomesan. Beijing Medical Journal, 1979, 1(1): 25-26. (In Chinese)

21. Garcia HH, DelBrutto OH. Nash TE, et al. New concepts in the diagnosis and management of neu-rocysticercosis (Taeniasolium). Am J Trop Med Hyg, 2005, 72(1): 3-9.

22. Ali BH. A short review of some pharmacological, therapeutic and toxicological properties of praziquantel in man and animals. Pak J Pharm Sci, 2006, 19 (2): 170-175.

23. Zhang DC. Series of Traditional Chinese Medicine, Traditional Chinese Medical Parasitology. Shaanxi science and technology press, 1998, 108-140. (In Chinese)

24. Feng LZ. Study on the treatment of tapeworm with pumpkin seeds and areca. Natl Med J China, 1956, 42(02): 138-147.

1.2.2.2 Cysticercosis

Cysticercosis is a parasitic disease caused by ingesting the eggs of the pork tapeworm, *T. solium*. Human tapeworm infection (teniasis) occurs after ingesting raw or undercooked pork, and cysticercosis occurs after the ingestion of *T. solium* eggs. Cysticercus is also called swine cysticercus; it is the young form of the pork tapeworm. Cysticercus can parasitize a human's muscle, brain, eye, or heart, and cause cysticercosis, which has serious consequences. The earliest tapeworms were recorded in the works of ancient Egyptians in 2000 BC.

Cysticercus are vesicular, white, translucent, about 10 mm × 5 mm in size, have a thin wall, a capsule filled cyst fluid, and a small grain size of white spots, including the head of the rolled section. In the first section, in addition to four suction cups, they also have rostellum and hooks. Even visible deformity is orbserved in the first section, the number of suckers can be 2–7, and can be a double-top projections, as well as the number of small hooks which is also different. Cysticerci size and shape may be affected by the parasite's location, condition, and nutrition.

Epidemiology

Aristotle's (384–322 BC) description of pork measles attributes pork infection with tapeworm to ancient Greece. This is one of the reasons that pork is forbidden by Jewish and Islamic dietary laws. Recent examination of the evolutionary histories of hosts and parasites, as well as DNA evidence, show that ancestors of modern humans in Africa became exposed to tapeworm (and then passed the infection on to domestic animals) when they scavenged for food and bovidae more than 10,000 years ago.

Johannes Udalric Rumler described cysticercosis in 1555. However, the connection between tapeworms and cysticercosis was not recognized at that time. Friedrich Küchenmeister fed pork-containing cysticerci of *T. solium* to humans awaiting execution in a prison around 1850. He discovered the developing and adult tapeworms in their intestines after they had been executed. By mid-19th century, it was established that cysticercosis was caused by the ingestion of *T. solium* eggs.

Solid lumps between one and two centimeters may develop under the skin in some cases, particularly in Asian populations. These lumps can become painful and swollen, and then resolve after months or years. Neurological symptoms can be caused by a specific form called neurocysticercosis. This is one of the most common causes of seizures in patients living in developing countries.

The highest numbers of cysticercosis infections are found among humans who live close to pigs. High prevalence rates are reported in Latin America, Mexico, West Africa, Russia, Pakistan, India, Southeast Asia, and Northeast China. The frequency of infections has decreased due to better hygiene, better sanitation of facilities, and stricter meat inspection regulations in developed countries. In China, the cysticerco-sis infection rate is estimated to be 0.14–3.2% in humans, with approximately three million people infected.[1] Worldwide deaths from cysticercosis were about 1,200 in 2010.[2]

Diagnosis

Aspiration of a cyst is a good diagnosis of cysticercosis. Taking pictures of the brain with magnetic resonance imaging (MRI) or computer tomography (CT) are most useful for the diagnosis of cysticercosis in the brain. Suspected patients will also be asked about his/her symptoms, travel history, and kinds of foods consumed, which all help in the diagnosis of cysticercosis. If a person has been diagnosed with cysticercosis, his/her family members should also be tested for intestinal tapeworm infection. Please refer to the teniasis section above for more information on intestinal tapeworm infections.

Immunological diagnosis

- Detection of circulating antibodies: It uses a known antigen to detect unknown antibody *in vivo* in patients, however, the cysticercus antigen composition is very complex. Different strains of insects and even different stages of the same insect strains are antigenically different, and with a variety of parasites, especially with hydatid the presence of common antigen.
- Detection of circulating antigens: The body will produce corresponding anti-bodies if a human is infected with cysticerci. The antibodies will remain in the body for a long time, sometimes even more than 10 years. Therefore, the tested antibodies can only confirm that the body has been infected with cyst-icerci. They cannot serve as a basis for current patients and cannot determine

efficacy of treatment. The half-life of circulating anti-parasite secretions or principle metabolite is short; therefore, the circulating antigen shows the presence of live cysticerci. For the detection of circulating antigen, an anti-cysticercosis antigen monoclonal antibody must be first prepared. There are many ways to carry out the circulating antigen assay, including but not limited to the reverse hemagglutination and double antibody sandwich ELISA. These are sensitive, specific, reliable, and simple, and are especially suitable for grassroots applications. With an excess of circulating antigen, the antigen and antibody form circulating immune complexes, as the antigen binding clusters occupied with the detection limit of the applied antibody binding, thus affecting the detection of circulating antigen.

Common immunodiagnostics

The common immunodiagnostics for cysticercosis are described below:

- CF: This is a classic test, and was the first immunodiagnostic technique used for the diagnosis of cysticercosis. It does not require any purification of antigens and antibodies, or any special equipment. It was widely used before the 1970s.
- ID: Another early immunological diagnostic method, with high sensitivity. However, it is usually affected by antigenic cross-reactivity, and after a while, it still comes up positive responses even when the parasites are killed. Due to its ease of use and high sensitivity, it is still used for sieving, and remains the simple method for epidemiological investigation.
- LA: This is a test using polystyrene latex sensitized immunodiagnostics with a cysticercus antigen or antibody. It is simple, fast, easy to spread, and suitable for grassroots use.
- Immunofluorescent Assay (IFA): IFA is applied to a fluorescent dye immune response. The advantage is that the preparation of a fluorescent-labeled antibody can be used for a variety of antigen/antibody screening systems, and it can measure unknown antigens or antibodies.
- HA: HA is simple to operate, requires no special equipment, the sensitivity is good, and it suitable for field and primary use for the wider application

of current methods. The disadvantages are poor reproducibility between batches and individual differences, and sensitized red blood cells do not keep their deficiencies. The effect of a purified antigen is significantly better than that of a crude antigen.

- Enzyme immunoassay (EIA) or ELISA: The EIA technique has been widely used, and on this basis, has developed into a variety of diagnostic tests.

Imaging diagnosis

X-ray, CT, and MRI can be used for the diagnosis of cerebral cysticercosis. As the parasitic cysticerci can be found in parts of the brain at different stages of development, their shape, size, and surroundings do not yield the same reaction. Cysticercus brain parenchyma are round, similar in size (4–5 mm in diameter), and surrounded by mild inflammation, edema, and mild gliosis. Intraventricular cysticercus immerses in the cerebrospinal fluid, therefore producing larger parasites, up to 3–4 cm in diameter; it can cause meningitis and ependymal obstructive hydrocephalus. Cysticerci which invade the brain tissue due to early-stage parasites are too small to absorb the same value and cannot be identified on CT. They are visible at different times at different degrees of enhancement of the lesion. If a large number of cysticerci gets into the brain, this can cause acute meningitis, cerebral edema, and intracranial hypertension. Cysticerci death can release a variant protein, and can also cause acute inflammation, edema, intracranial hypertension, or brain abscesses.

The electroencephalogram (EEG) differs in patients with cerebral cysticercosis. In patients with neurocysticercosis, the EEG changes the severity of symptoms, with their degree not always consistent. An EEG abnormality rate is about 1/3–1/2 of the total number of patients. EEG abnormalities are mainly mild and moderate, more diffuse changes, no characteristic pattern is observed with the central nervous system EEG, however, the EEG may reflect brain function in patients with neurocysticercosis. EEG is consistent with the development of the disease; if the disease improves, the EEG gradually goes to normal.

Treatment

In recent years, the application of praziquantel and benzimidazole has played a significant role in the treatment of cysticercosis and dissemination via blocking.

Praziquantel is a broad-spectrum anthelmintic used to treat human cysticercosis. Praziquantel increases the permeability of cell membranes for calcium ions resulting in parasite paralysis and contracture. Blood free of praziquantel can flow freely through the blood-brain barrier, cerebrospinal fluid concentrations of blood concentration of 1/7–1/5 can achieve an effective insecticide concentration. After oral absorption via the gastrointestinal tract, peak plasma concentrations are reached 1.5–2 hours later. Due to the highly fat-soluble composition of the drug, it is quickly distributed in the human tissue and combines with about 80-85% bound to plasma proteins. Within 24 hours of it being administered, 90% of the drug is excreted by the kidneys.

The usual dose is 50 mg/kg body weight administered orally three times daily, for up to nine days. This results in 60–70% of brain parenchymal cysticercosis lesions disappearing. If necessary, a course of treatment can be repeated a month after the fist treatment. According to praziquantel's pharmacokinetic characteristics, after two hours of administration, peak plasma concentrations decrease rapidly. If the dose is changed to every two hours once daily, there may be high concentrations of praziquantel in the blood for up to 12 hours, and two hours after the previous prevents blood concentration decline. Serving twice as cimetidine can increase plasma concentrations of praziquantel. Praziquantel does not need to be absorbed metabolically. In the half-life of praziquantel, it can quickly penetrate into the cerebrospinal fluid and into the worm slowly. *In vitro*, about 1 mg/L concentration of praziquantel can destroy the tapeworm, but due to the barrier between the fluid and the cerebrospinal fluid of the cysticerci, drug concentration in the brain parenchyma needs to be increased 7–10 times in order to effectively kill cysticercosis.

Albendazole is a novel broad-spectrum anthelmintic. It is 85% effective for treating cysticercosis, and it has fewer side effects. Its mechanism of action may be related to the inhibition of the parasite and inhibition of glycogen absorption of antifumarate reductase.

There is no uniform regimen for the use of albendazole. Experiments show that albendazole is effective at a single dose of 50 mg/kg body weight. Currently, the treatment of cerebral cysticercosis is usually a daily dose of 15 mg/kg body weight. Twice daily dosages are appropriate. It has been proved that taking the drug for eight days or even as little as three days will achieve the desired effect. In a parenchymal-type patient, a dose of 15 mg/kg body weight daily for eight days results in 80-85% of the encapsulation disappearing.

Albendazole is also effective in the treatment of eye and ventricular cysticerci, especially for large subarachnoid and spinal cysticercosis. After treatment, cysticercus nodules harden, shrink, and finally disappear. Fatty diets can promote the absorption of albendazole. Enteral neutral fat can make bile secretion, promoting the absorption of the drug by the action of bile acids.

After the lesions caused by live cysticerci can be completely absorbed through early treatment, there is no sequela left; but in case of late treatment of lesions, there is no total absorption. It has been reported that in 41.7% of patients treated with albendazole, brain lesions are absorbed within six months. Early-stage infection, short course of young stage encephalitis, a large amount of the drug (25 mg/kg per day of body weight), and long course of medication (20 days) all contribute to the drug having positive effects.

Anti-inflammatory treatment of neurocysticercosis: The host immune response is a major cause of complications due to cerebral cysticercosis. Because of immune tolerance, long-term survival of cysticerci in the brain causes only mild or no symptom, while some patients have a strong immune response, resulting in edema around the lesion or fiber of vasculitis. Nervous system damage, and the extent of the immune response and the prognosis is directly related to the host, rather than being the result of direct damage caused by cysticerci.

Corticosteroids are effective anti-inflammatory drugs used to treat encephalitis and cysticercus parasites if patients have a necrosis-induced inflammatory response. These reactions are common in children and young women, but are rare in adults. To control cerebral edema, a short course of high-dose intravenous dexamethasone or methyl prednisolone may be used. An immunosuppressant azathioprine may also be added. If a patient has encephalitis and mitigation of high intracranial pressure before anti-cysticercus treatment, a 2–3-day praziquantel treatment may be administered. If there is an adverse reaction, dexamethasone can be given for two to three days, which is usually sufficient to control these reactions. Dexamethasone can increase the plasma concentrations of albendazole; therefore, four days before treatment, a daily dose of 10–20 mg can be given.[3]

Control strategy

In 1992, the International Task Force for Disease Eradication reported that cysticercosis is potentially eradicable, as there are no animal reservoirs besides humans and pigs. Humans are the only definitive hosts and harbor the adult *T. solium* worms, whereas both humans and pigs can act as intermediate hosts (that is, eggs from human feces are transmitted to other humans or pigs).

Theoretically, it is easy to break the life cycle by targeting interventions to various stages of the life cycle. These include: improving sanitation, massive chemotherapy of infected individuals, and educating people on how to stop the cycle. Freezing pork or cooking it and inspecting meat are effective methods to cease the life cycle of *T. solium*. Treating pigs or vaccinating them is another possible intervention. The pig industry has developed rapidly and most pigs were housed post-World War II in Western European countries. Due to this, pig cysticercosis has largely been eliminated in those regions.

Particular attention should be paid to preventing contamination by water, and by eating vegetables and eggs. Worm vaccination is expected to become a powerful tool for the prevention of cysticercosis. A variety of parasite antigens for vaccination could protect swine against cysticercosis. However, due to the direct production of antigen by the parasite, its quantity and quality cannot be ensured, limiting the application of this vaccine. Preparing the tapeworm antigen from other insect species could become an alternative, widespread vaccine antigen. A recombinant antigen will help overcome difficulties in antigen sources.

References

1. Wu W, Qian X, Huang Y. A review of the control of *Clonorchiasis sinensis* and *Taenia solium* taeniasis/cysticercosis in China. Parasitol Res, 2012, 111(5): 1879-1884.

2. Maurice J. Of pigs and people–WHO prepares to battle cysticercosis. Lancet, 2014, 384(9943): 571-572.

3. Murrell K D, Dorny P, Flisser A, et al. WHO/FAO/OIE guidelines for the surveillance, prevention and control of taeniosis/cysticercosis. 2005, 27-43.

1.2.3 Cryptosporidiosis

Tyzzer was the first scientist to find *Cryptosporidium* spp. in the gastric epithelial cells of mice. In 1976, Nime reported that people could also be infected with *Cryptosporidium* spp., which resulted in people paying more attention on it.

Cryptosporidium spp. is a kind of protist and belongs to the apicomplexa. At present, there are more than 27 known species of *Cryptosporidium* and more than 40 genotypes. Nearly 20 species can infect humans, however, most infections are attributed to *Cryptosporidium hominis* and *C. parvum*; *C. hominis* is human specific species, while *C. parvum* is zoonotic one.

The whole life cycle of *Cryptosporidium* spp. occurs in only one host, known as the endogenous stage, and includes asexual reproduction, sexual reproduction and spore reproduction. The fecal oocyst discharged by the host is infectious. After ingested by the host, the infectious oocysts release sporozoites which can attach to the microvilli of small intestinal epithelial cells and then enter the cells. In the parasitophorous vacuole located between intracellular and extracytoplasmic, the multiple fission of asexual reproduction (schizogony) takes place. The sporozoites grow into trophozoites first and develop into Type I meronts after three nuclear divisions. Every mature Type I meront contains six or height merozoites, which can invade intestinal epithelial cells after released and become Type II meronts after two nuclear divisions. The four merozoites of each mature Type II meront can also invade intestinal epithelial cells and become macrogamonts and microgamonts, the female and male sexual forms (gametogony), respectively. In the stage of sexual reproduction, the female gametophyte develops into female gamete, while the male gametophyte produces 16 male gametes. The zygotes, formed by male and female gametes, develop into oocysts through spore reproduction. There are two types of oocysts, thin-walled and thick-walled. Twenty percent thin-walled oocysts can release the sporozoite to reinfect the host and start asexual reproduction again. Others are thick-walled oocysts and they sporulate in the host cell or the lumen. The sporulated oocysts are infective upon being excreted with host feces. The entire life cycle usually takes 5–11 days.

Epidemiology

Cryptosporidium oocysts transmit to a new host via the fecal-oral route through contact with contaminated water or uncooked food. Drinking water polluted by infective feces is an important way to transmit oocysts and has become a serious public health problem. In addition, people can become infected through contact body with recreational water, such as swimming pools, containing oocysts.

Cryptosporidiosis, also known as crypto, is caused by *Cryptosporidium* infection. It generally occurs 2–14 days after infection, with symptoms including watery diarrhea, abdominal cramps, low-grade fever, nausea, vomiting, weight loss, and so on. These symptoms often last 1–3 weeks and clear without treatment in immunocompetent hosts, however, they are particularly severe and may be fatal in immunocompromised individuals such as acquired immune deficiency syndrome (AIDS) patients. In addition, in young children, especially malnourished ones, the diarrhea caused by cryptosporidiosis can be extensive and leads to high mortality. In fact, *Cryptosporidium* has become the second major cause (after rotavirus) of diarrhea in children aged below five years in developing countries.

Cryptosporidiosis is distributed all over the world; it has been found in more than 90 countries. The average infection rate of the population is 1–3% in Europe and North America, 5% in Asia, and up to 10% in Africa. Early studies show that the *Cryptosporidium* infection rate was 5–10% in developing countries and 1% in developed countries among immunocompetent individuals. However, with the application of polymerase chain reaction (PCR) and other molecular biological detection techniques, the infection rate is significantly higher than earlier reports which indicated the current *Cryptosporidium* infections are still underestimated.

In 1987, Han Fan found that people were infected with *Cryptosporidium* in Nanjing, the first time to discover such infection in China. Cryptosporidiosis was found in some parts of China afterwards. Epidemiological data show that there are cryptosporidiosis patients in at least 17 provinces, with the infection rate between 1.4–10.4%.[1] In 2000, Lu Shaohong et al. found 548 cases of children with diarrhea in the Zhejiang Province, with the rate of *Cryptosporidium* infection at 10.4%. Cheng Yongzhang et al. reported that the infection rate among humans in Hangzhou was 8.7% in 2000. In 2001, through the microscopic examination of 5,421 stool samples from different populations of 11 cities in Anhui Province, Li Chaopin et al. found that the infection rate was 1.33%, and that infected persons were usually young children, adult diarrhea patients, and immunocompromised persons. Cai Ru et al. reported that the infection rate in the diarrhea population was 5.6% in Huainan area in 2003. In a survey of 500 feces samples belonging to different groups in Luwan District, Shanghai, in 2005, Zhou Hongfang et al. found that the infection rate was 4.8%. Among them, the infection rate was 5.30% in patients with diarrhea, 13.33% in residents with dogs, and 0% in community residents. Yin Jianhai et al. detected 947 cases of diarrhea patients in Shanghai in 2012 and found that the infection rate was 0.31%, indicating that the infection rate is low in urban area.

Control strategy

Water contaminated with oocysts is an important vehicle for the transmission of *Cryptosporidium*. Chlorine disinfectant, a usual reagent, is not applicable to control *Cryptosporidium* in drinking water, as the oocysts, which have hard and thick walls, are highly resistant to it and its inactivity needs very high concentrations of chlorine disinfectant and a long contact time. Standard water filtration may not be sufficient to eliminate *Cryptosporidium* either and a filter with an aperture size of less than one micrometer is needed. Slow sand filters, diatomaceous earth filters, or other cartridge filters that can remove *Cryptosporidium,* specifically can remove 99% of oocysts. The most reliable way to purify potable water from potential contamination is to boil it for at least 1–3 minutes at an altitude of 2,000 meters. Ultraviolet light is also effective in inactivating *Cryptosporidium* and only low doses are required.

The best way to prevent *Cryptosporidium* infection is to have good health habits. People should avoid eating uncooked food or drinking raw water that is possibly contaminated. Hands should be washed carefully after any situation that may have put someone in contact with oocysts, such as going to the bathroom or disposing of animal feces. Patients with cryptosporidiosis should not swim in public pools for at least two weeks after their diarrhea stops, as the oocysts may still be shedding for a while and reside in the anal and genital areas. Immunocompromised people, in particular, should be very careful in communal water areas.

At present, there is no specific therapy for cryptosporidiosis. Because cryptosporidiosis is self-limiting in immunocompetent individuals, the general treatment is improving immunity. The common method is oral or intravenous rehydration of glucose, sodium bicarbonate, and potassium, and replacement of electrolytes. For children with severe malnutrition and immunocompromised individuals, especially HIV/AIDS patients with severe diarrhea, active, supporting treatment is necessary.

Currently, the common therapeutic drug to treat cryptosporidiosis is nitazoxanide. Nitazoxanide, a type of thiazolidine compound, has a broad anti-parasitic spectrum and was approved to treat cryptosporidiosis as the first specialized drug by the Food and Drug Administration of the United States (US FDA) in 2002. Nitazoxanide is feasible for patients aged one year or older. A clinical trial showed that nitazoxanide has good efficacy in adults and children without HIV, and can significantly reduce mortality among children with malnutrition. The treatment duration is about 3–14 days, and the oral doses are 500 mg twice daily for adults and adolescents, 200 mg twice daily for children aged 4–11 years, and 100 mg twice daily for children aged one to three years.[2] Unfortunately, nitazoxanide has not yet been found to be effective against HIV-infected people.

A wide range of available drugs have been tested to treat *Cryptosporidium* infections in immunocompetent patients. Paromomycin can ameliorate cryptosporidiosis in patients with AIDS. It is also effective in children with cryptosporidiosis, but the response is significantly lower than what it is for nitazoxanide.[3] Improving immune function in immunocompromised hosts is the key for preventing cryptosporidiosis; immunotherapy, such as combination antiretroviral therapy, may be effective in AIDS patients.[4]

Diagnosis

The diagnostic methods used to detect cryptosporidiosis include microscopy, staining, antibody detection, and so on. Oocysts in feces can be identified with the help of microscopy, and at least three fecal samples are needed to ensure accuracy. Fecal samples can be concentrated by many ways, including modified formalin-ethyl acetate concentration, modified zinc sulfate centrifugal flotation, and Sheather's sugar flotation. The *Cryptosporidium* oocyst is very tiny and difficult to distinguish by microscopy directly, but the resolution can be markedly improved by using fluorescent microscopy. Staining techniques include auramine staining, modified acid-fast staining, etc. Auramine staining is available for fresh or formalin fixed samples, with the oocysts showing up as bright, white, round, yellow-green fluorescent after staining. The modified acid-fast staining is most reliable and used to detect oocysts traditionally. In this method, the oocysts are stained red, which leads to difficulties in distinguishing the oocysts and to many red acid particles in fecal samples. To improve the detection rate, fecal samples can be stained with auramine first and then again using the modified acid-fast staining method: oocyst forms are the same as in the acid-fast staining, while nonspecific particles appear blue-black.

Detecting antigens is another way to diagnose cryptosporidiosis. These include direct fluorescent antibody (dFA) test, ELISA, and PCR. Direct fluorescent antibody has high sensitivity and specificity, but cannot distinguish species and genotypes. ELISA, with a high degree of automation, can screen a large number of samples in a short time. Polymerase chain reaction can identify the specific species of *Cryptosporidium*, but cannot distinguish the vitality and infectivity of the oocysts, as oocyst DNA can be preserved for at least a week after cell death. The viability of oocysts can be determined by detecting and amplifying a viable excysted sporozoite DNA fragment using the PCR method.

Drug discovery

Cryptosporidium invades the host and starts its life cycle in the small intestine epithelial cells. Therefore, orally administered drugs absorbed locally in the intestine will be effective. The reproduction and growth of *Cryptosporidium* completely occurs in epithelial cells, thereby drugs have to pass through the membrane of cells and parasitophorous vacuole first to work. However, in immunodeficient hosts, the *Cryptosporidium* infection can be more widely distributed, finding its way into the bile vessel, pancreatic duct, stomach, esophagus, and even respiratory tract. Systemic drug absorption is thus essential. The endogenous stage of *Cryptosporidium* can be achieved *in vitro* by several different cell lines. Although it is difficult to capture the entire life cycle by the current methods, it also contributes to screening for new drugs to treat cryptosporidiosis.

Screening of drugs or compounds that have been developed is another way of finding anti-*Cryptosporidium* agents. After the identification of potential lead compounds by cell-based screening in compound libraries *in vitro*, further studies *in vivo* are required. For example, 727 compounds were tested for activity on parasite growth in HCT-8 epithelial cells, yielding 16 confirmed selective inhibitors, including 3-hydroxy-3-methylglutaryl-coenzyme A (HMG-CoA) reductase inhibitors. HMG-CoA reductase is necessary for the *de novo* synthesis of isoprenoids. However, *Cryptosporidium* lacks the enzymes required to synthesize the isoprenoid precursors and need the help of the host's cells to achieve it, so that inhibitors of the critical enzymes can block the growth of parasite.[5]

With more and more researches being conducted on *Cryptosporidium*, designing new compounds aimed at specific targets, especially indispensable and unique ones, is another way to develop drugs to treat cryptosporidiosis. *Cryptosporidium* lacks the genes for *de novo* biosynthesis of amino acids, nucleotides, and sugars, while many metabolism-related genes also have been lost, including the mitochondrial respiratory chain, apicoplast pathways, and so on. Thus, *Cryptosporidium* must rely heavily on salvaging nutrients from the host to maintain its normal metabolism. Because these metabolic pathways are absent in the host or greatly different from the host's, many of the enzymes have opportunities to become the potential drug targets.

Calcium-dependent protein kinase 1 (CDPK1), a unique protein kinase in *Cryptosporidium* and other apicomplexan parasites, plays an important role in the process of cell invasion by mediating calcium signals.[6] Inhibitors of CDPK1 can block CDPK1's function and ultimately kill the *Cryptosporidium* cell. Structural analysis shows that glycine, as a gatekeeper residue, in the adenosine triphosphate (ATP) binding site of CDPK1, makes a hydrophobic region more available for inhibitors active against *Cryptosporidium*. Pyrazolopyrimidine derivatives have exhibited anti-*Cryptosporidium* activity both *in vitro* and in mouse infection models.[6]

Clan CA (papain-like) cysteine proteases, which are structurally different with analogous enzymes in humans and associated with excystation and host cell invasion, may be another potential target against cryptosporidiosis. The selective protease inhibitor K11777 (N-methyl-piperazine-Phe-homoPhe-vinylsulfone phenyl) has shown anti-*Cryptosporidium* activity both *in vitro* and *in vivo*.[7]

Another potential drug target is oxidoreductase inosine 5'-monophosphate dehydrogenase (IMPDH), which can catalyze the conversion of inosine-5'-monophosphate into xanthosine-5'-monophosphate in the process of guanine nucleotide biosynthesis. *Cryptosporidium* cannot synthesize purine nucleotides *de novo*, thus it has to absorb adenosines from the host and convert them into guanine nucleotides via a pathway involving IMPDH. The structure of IMPDH is different in *Cryptosporidium* and humans, and a series of inhibitors for this enzyme have been found. Many derivatives of urea, benzoxazole, and benzopyrano [4, 3-c] pyrazole exhibit inhibitory activity of IMPDH at low concentrations and some of them exhibit anti-*C. parvum* activity. Peptides have also been investigated as IMPDH inhibitors. The phylomer peptides, identified in a yeast two-hybrid screening, have shown inhibitory activity of IMPDH *in vitro*, and several of them have anti-*Cryptosporidium* ability.[8]

Much research has been conducted on other targets. *Cryptosporidium* depends on glycolysis to produce ATP, further producing lactate, ethanol, and acetate, thus the inhibition of hexokinase and lactate dehydrogenase is effective against the parasite. *Cryptosporidium* contains a bi-functional thymidylate synthase-dihydrofolate reductase, a key enzyme in the folate biosynthesis pathway, and compounds aimed at this enzyme show conspicuous anti-*Cryptosporidium* activity *in vitro*. Fatty acyl-coenzyme A synthetase, which exists in the parasitophorus vacuole membrane, is essential for the fatty acid metabolism of *Cryptosporidium*. It can be inhibited by Triacsin C significantly *in vitro*, with *C. parvum* oocyst production shown to reduce by 88% in mice.[9]

Additionally, the development of a vaccine is a feasible way to prevent cryptosporidiosis. Several antigens are being developed as candidates, such as profilin, Cp15, Gp60, P2 antigen, Muc4, Muc5, and *Cryptosporidium* apyrase.[4]

Cryptosporidiosis, as a category of neglected tropical diseases (NTDs), mainly affects underdeveloped countries and areas characterized by poor hygiene. Recently, more and more evidence has shown that cryptosporidiosis may become a serious problem among children and immunodeficient persons. As there is no specific treatment for cryptosporidiosis, studies mostly focus on the development of novel therapeutics. Although there have been already a lot of advancements, no new drug or vaccine has been approved for use to treat cryptosporidiosis clinically. Challenges still exist and more efforts should therefore be paid to this disease.

References

1. Lv S, Tian LJ, Liu Q, et al. Water-related parasitic diseases in China. Int J Environ Res Public Health, 2013, 10(5): 1977-2016.

2. Miyamoto Y, Eckmann L. Drug development against the major diarrhea-causing parasites of the small intestine, *Cryptosporidium* and *Giardia*. Frontiers Microbiol, 2015, 6: 1208.

3. Sparks H, Nair G, Castellanos-Gonzalez A, et al. Treatment of *Cryptosporidium*: what we know, gaps, and the way forward. Curr Trop Med Rep, 2015, 2(3): 181-187.

4. Checkley W, White AC Jr., Jaganath D, et al. A review of the global burden, novel diagnostics, therapeutics, and vaccine targets for Cryptosporidium. Lancet Infect Dis, 2015, 15(1): 85-94.

5. Bessoff K, Sateriale A, Lee KK, et al. Drug repurposing screen reveals FDA-approved inhibitors of human HMG-CoA reductase and isoprenoid synthesis that block *Cryptosporidium parvum* growth. Antimicrob Agents Chemother, 2013, 57(4): 1804-1814.

6. Castellanos-Gonzalez A, White AC Jr, Ojo K K, et al. A novel calcium-dependent protein kinase inhibitor as a lead compound for treating cryptosporidiosis. J Infect Dis, 2013, 208(8): 1342-1348.

7. Ndao M, Nath-Chowdhury M, Sajid M, et al. A cysteine protease inhibitor rescues mice from a lethal *Cryptosporidium parvum* infection. Antimicrob Agents Chemother, 2013, 57(12): 6063-6073.

8. Jefferies R, Yang R, Woh CK, et al. Target validation of the inosine monophosphate dehydrogenase (IMPDH) gene in *Cryptosporidium* using Phylomer(®) peptides. Exp Parasitol, 2015, 148: 40-48.

9. Guo F, Zhang H, Fritzler JM, et al. Amelioration of *Cryptosporidium parvum* infection in vitro and in vivo by targeting parasite fatty acyl-coenzyme A synthetases. J Infect Dis, 2014, 209(8): 127-1287.

1.3 Vector-borne parasitic diseases

Vector-borne parasitic diseases are a group of important diseases transmitted through vectors. They include: (i) dengue fever, malaria, lymphatic filariasis, etc., spread by mosquitoes; (ii) leishmaniasis spread by species of *Lutzomyia* spp.; and (iii) rickettsia, human babesiosis, etc., spread by ticks. China has a vast territory with rich vector resources which are likely to cause vector-borne parasitic diseases. These kinds of infectious diseases account for 5–10% of the total number of infectious diseases in China annually, but the death toll from them accounts for 30–40% of the total deaths caused by infectious diseases.

On the other hand, due to globalization, the status of global health security is becoming fragile. For instance, there is a rapid occurrence of cross-border transmission of infectious diseases, with more domestic infectious diseases spreading to other countries. A report from the American Medical Association that analyzed eight main causes of infectious diseases showed that the top one was an increasing of population travel, as such, the pathogens and vectors are carried by people from one country to another. Frequent migration of populations and vectors makes the traditional way of disease isolation impossible. This can also easily cause an outbreak of infectious diseases in a country and spread rapidly to other areas. Therefore, a particular attention needs to be paid to vector-borne parasitic diseases, including lymphatic filariasis transmitted by mosquitoes, leishmaniasis transmitted by sand fly, and human babesiosis transmitted by ticks, especially with the development of globalization.

1.3.1　Lymphatic filariasis

Worldwide, more than 80 million people are at risk of lymphatic filariasis (LF). Its clinical features are mainly acute lymphangitis and lymphadenitis, as well as chronic lymphatic obstruction and resulting symptoms such as elephantiasis crus, hydrocele, chyluria, and so on. There are no obvious symptoms, except for blood microfilaria, the so-called "filarial infection". These filarial microfilariae have more stringent characteristics and appear in the peripheral blood flow at night.[1] *Wuchereria bancrofti* and *Brugia malayi* are the two main causative agents of lymphatic filariasis in humans.

Adult worms are slim, white, slightly pointed at both ends, with a smooth surface, and are dioecious. They often entangle together, and often detected in a number of three to five adult worms in one part of the human lymphatic system. The *Wuchereria bancrofti* worm is 28–42 mm in length and 0.1 mm in width; the length and width of the female are about double of that of the male. The *Brugia malayi* worm is shorter. *Brugia malayi* and *W. bancrofti* females are similar and their internal structures are almost identical, while there are very small differences in the male worm. The life expectancy of adult worm is estimated at 10–15 years.[3]

Lymphatic filariasis was a widely distributed epidemic in China. Almost 1,000 counties/cities in 16 provinces/autonomous regions/municipalities reported LF patients in the 1950s. According to the pre-control survey results, in the 1980s, there were 30 million filariasis-infected people in China, of which 25 million had micro-filaremia and 5.4 million had chronic filariasis. More than 300 million people were at risk of getting the disease. Since 1949, when the People's Republic of China (P.R. China) was founded, the government supported a total of 72 million blood tests for LF, treating 210 million person-times. The average detection rate of microfilariae in the population reduced from 5.66% in 1950s to 0.001% in 1994, and 864 epidemic counties and cities reached the level of basically eliminating filariasis. In 2006, the country submitted *China's National Report on Lymphatic Filariasis Elimination* to the Fourth Global Alliance for the Elimination of Lymphatic Filariasis, which was approved by the WHO on May 9, 2007.[4]

Epidemiology

In the 1950s, 864 counties/cities in 16 provinces/autonomous regions/municipalities including Shandong, Henan, Hubei, Anhui, Jiangsu, Shanghai, Zhejiang, Jiangxi, Fujian, Guangdong, Hainan, Hunan, Guangxi, Guizhou, Sichuan, and Chongqing, reported LF patients. Bancroftian filariasis was epidemic in 463 counties/cities and brugian filariasis in 217 counties/cities.

Among the endemic counties in 1950s, about 4% were hyper-epidemic areas (microfilaria rate >20%), 31% were middle-epidemic areas (microfilaria rate between 5–20%), and about 65% were hypoendemic areas (microfilaria rate ≤5%).[9]

In the 1980s, there were more than 300 million threatened people with approxi-mately 30 million case reports. From the total number of patients, more than two-thirds had bancroftian filariasis.[5]

Risk factor analyses of LF prevalence were conducted taking into account the economy, hygienic conditions, human behavior and living habits, geographical envi-ronment, species of mosquito vector, and species of filariae. In epidemic areas, poor economic and sanitary conditions were found to induce higher prevalence rates.[6]

Control strategy

Stage 1: From the 1950s to the 1960s, the focus was on eliminating the source of infection. It was generally believed that the control of LF should be based on the elimination of the infection source, integrated with the control of mosquito vectors. In 1950s, the WHO also advocated for a comprehensive strategy to control LF such as control the vectors and have more personal protection from biting. [7] In theory, the effect of integrated control should be better, but as it requires large human and material resources, this may not be the case in reality.

The prevalence of LF in China was widespread and comprehensive, which made the control difficult. In the early 1960s, Chinese scholars investigated a control strategy based on the pathogenic biological characteristics of LF, such as: (i) filarial larvae is only developed in the mosquito and does not reproduce for the next generation; (ii) the mosquito infection period from filarial larvae entering into the mosquito body to appear dominant infection by a variety of factors; (iii) in China, neither of the two species of LF have a reservoir host, with anti-filariasis drugs such as diethyl-carbamazine (DEC; also called hetrazan) were affirmed to have high efficacy in treatment. The same study showed that continuous use of the single drug (hetrazan) against LF for 10 years could significantly reduce the disease prevalence from 10% to 0.8%. [14] Therefore, mass chemotherapy was the most important intervention to control LF at the time. The pilot of the comparative study found that there was no significant difference in effectiveness between implementation of a comprehensive control approach and a single source of eradication approach, with both strategies able to decrease the microfilaria rate to a relatively low level. However, the cost of the comprehensive control approach was much higher.

A single hetrazan treatment was conducted in the 1950s to eliminate the source of infection, with the microfilaria rate reducing from 10.53% to 0.79% on average, by comparing the data from 1951 to 1957. After treatment had stopped for 12 years, the microfilaria rate was kept at a level of 0.42% in 1969, and then showed a downward trend without a rebound. This demonstrated that a single approach for eliminating sources of infection is able to achieve a microfilaria rate of less than 1% even after a period of consolidation time, such like five or ten years after mass chemotherapy. As a result in stage 2 (1960s–1970s), from 1971 to 1973, this approach was scaled up in various areas of the country. By the late 1970s, the strategy of eliminating sources of infection was implemented on a wide scale, leading to the elimination of LF in many parts of the country.

Stage 2: From the 1960s to the 1970s, large-scale treatment of hetrazan was implemented. In the 1950s, many clinical and field observations were made on the dosages and course of treatment with hetrazan against *B. malayi* and *W. bancrofti*. From the 1960s to the early 1970s, experiments were carried out for hetrazan treatment at community levels to control filariasis transmission. Results showed that the prevalence of LF is easy to reduce with this easy-to-operate approach, and the adverse events are very rare. A total of three schemes were undertaken to combat filariasis transmission using large-scale hetrazan treatment:[8]

- Repeated examination of microfilaremia: Conducting blood tests for the entire population in epidemic areas more than once, then treating infected individuals with hetrazan. This is early, commonly used in the prevention and treatment program, during 1965–1970, which was mainly used for *B. malayi* in low prevalence areas. The advantage of the approach is that it is relatively easy to implement, while the disadvantage is that blood tests easily miss the lesser density microfilaremia, pre-infection, and some patients cannot tolerate hetrazan and suffer from serious complications. No effective treatment is available for microfilaria in blood, therefore, this control strategy for *W. bancrofti* in highly endemic areas is often not ideal. [9]

- Repeated investigation and treatment provided in all epidemic villages: Besides treating patients that tested positive, those with a negative blood test were also given one course of hetrazan treatment. This program was a remedial measure to cure patients with low-density microfilaremia and also those who were still in the dominant pre-infection phase. Although this control effort was better and more consolidated, it still could not solve the problem of some patients not being able to tolerate hetrazan.[10]

- Using hetrazan-fortified salt: Hetrazan can kill a large number of microfilariae, but can then cause mild adverse events such as fever, headache, and nausea, etc. Therefore, it is difficult to implement hetrazan treatment among all patients in epidemic areas. The chemical formula of hetrazan is stable, which is resistant to high temperatures, undisturbed when mixing with foodstuffs, and its adverse effects such as fever, headache, and nausea are uncommon and mild. A pilot study conducted on using hetrazan-fortified salt was first carried out in China in the early 1970s in Shandong Province, achieving satisfactory results in this *W. bancrofti*-endemic province. When people had a daily intake of hetrazan-fortified salt, it reduces the dosage of hetrazan to about 50 mg per day; and this kind of low dosage can help have less adverse effects than people who take conventional doses. Before application, the hetrazan-fortified salt strategy was proven to be safe among three studied groups: (i) 61 patients with various inclusion disorders that should be banned for treatment with hetrazan; (ii) about 200 women who are pregnant or nursing with microfilaremia; and (iii) 234 newborns and infants. After the strategy was popularized in Shandong, it was applied in 13 other provinces and autonomous regions. A standardized hetrazan-fortified salt prevention and treatment program was then set up. The salt concentration was 0.3%, and the total amount of hetrazan per-capita intake at three, four, five, and six months was 4.5 g, 6 g, and 9 g, respectively. The plan could be altered to suit the local epidemic situation. The popularization and application of hetrazan-fortified salt greatly accelerated the pace of nation-wide control and elimination of filariasis.[11]

Stage 3: Investigating the threshold for filariasis transmission in the 1980s. What role does a low-density microfilaremia patient play in filariasis transmission? This is an important question when considering whether the prevention and control of filariasis can be consolidated and the goal of eliminating filariasis further realized. Chinese experts in filariasis epidemiology had been investigated this since the 1980s. According to a field survey, in the remaining microfilaremia, about 70% is of low-density (average five microfilariae/60 µL). In 1981 and 1982, five (one to eight microfilariae/60 µL) *B. malayi* cases and 87 (1–32 / 60 µL) *B. malayi* infected cases were observed at two pilot sites, with patients not getting treatment during the observation. All five cases of malayan filariasis were negative in the end of the study, all but two cases were positive. The infection rate of *W. bancrofti* dropped to zero and the frequency of *B. malayi* decreased to 0.03%. Two blood test surveys were conducted at each of the two surveillance sites, with no new infections detected. The results confirmed that the prevention and treatment of residual low-density micro-filaremia has no practical significance for the transmission of filariasis.

In 1982, China established the national filariasis transmission threshold research collaborative group. Twenty-one observation sites were set up according to different filarial and mosquito vectors, microfilariae, and microfilariae density in eleven provinces and autonomous regions. The treatment intervention was limited to these sites, with the goal of only observing the transmission patterns of filariasis in order to further understand the transmission threshold. The results showed that the threshold of filariasis transmitted in China in 1983 was of a low-density, the critical value of transmission of *B. malayi* was about 2.3% of population microfilariae, and the critical value of transmission of *W. bancrofti* in the population was about 1.7%. The thresholds of both species of filariae were below the critical value. The results of this study illustrated the low degree of filariasis transmission in China in the 1980s, which has theoretically and practically guided the design of the elimination program.[12]

Stage 4: Establishment of a vertical and horizontal monitoring system. In the early 1980s, as some areas gradually reached the goal of basically eliminating filariasis, monitoring the disease was put on the agenda. At that time, there was no theoretical guidance and practical experience relating to this. Through investigations on the transmission of filariasis at the late stage of prevention and treatment, researchers developed a monitoring strategy based on experience. It comprised: (i) residual microfilariae have no practical significance in the transmission of filariasis; and (ii) residual microfilaremia may gradually turn negative naturally with the time, which will achieve basic elimination of filariasis, and there will no longer be a need for blood screening and treatment; thus filariasis can be eliminated through systematic monitoring. On this basis, a unique vertical and horizontal filariasis monitoring system was established in China.[13]

The monitoring system comprises: (i) longitudinal monitoring: conducted in one epidemic area per locality (city, state), pathogenic, mosquito-borne, and serological surveillance are carried out continuously for the purpose of observing propagation dynamics and providing evidence for the elimination of filariasis; (ii) lateral monitoring: conducted in the epidemic counties and cities according to the original degree of prevalence and position in relation to the different administrative village sampling points, blood tests conducted among all in the county or city with patients treated in the remaining epidemic spots (administrative villages with a microfilaria rate higher than 1%); and (iii) floating population monitoring: the target is to live in the area and conduct etiological or serological surveillance of people from a prevalence area of filariasis for more than one epidemic season.[14]

The control objectives, standards, and methods of assessment were developed at the different stages of the control strategy. The objectives in the 1980s were basically to eliminate filariasis according to the requirements of the "Outline of the National Agricultural Development Plan (Draft)". After a long period of prevention and control practices and accumulation scientific evidences, it has been proposed to eliminate filariasis in China.

Based on the strategy of eliminating infection sources and taking into account all practical experiences, the standard for eliminating filariasis was formulated and promulgated by the Chinese Ministry of Health in 1983 with the following criteria: "all counties and cities that have a prevalence of filariasis must reduce the microfilaria positive rate at the administrative village level to below 1% after proper prevention and control".

As most of the provinces and autonomous regions have basically eliminated filariasis from 1983 onwards, what were the next targets? Whether eradicating filariasis should be proposed has become an urgent issue. In 1991, the target to eradicate filariasis in China was scientifically defined. Chinese experts proposed management theory and make the practice of prevention and control step by step. The epidemiological properties of less efficient transmission of filariasis by pathogenic biology have been demonstrated by studies on the threshold of filariasis transmission. For example, by the early 1990s, according to a series of longitudinal blood tests conducted at 82 longitudinal monitoring sites, there were more than 130,000 people and 203 residual microfilaremia patients in the country. A blood test was conducted among more than 8.89 million people across the country for horizontal monitoring. Although in some areas newly infected persons were detected, the population microfilaria rate, the mosquito infection rate, and the population serum antibody positive rate all showed a downward trend. A large number of monitoring results provide a practical basis for the formulation of the goal to eradicate filariasis. Scientifically, the elimination of filariasis refers to the elimination of the disease's source of infection, that is, curing microfilaremia (not including those who have no microfilariae but have pathological lesions), which will stop the spread of the filariasis epidemic.[15]

The Chinese Ministry of Health issued the "Standard for the Elimination of Filariasis (Trial Version)" in 1994. It was revised and officially released in 1996. It summarized the criteria for the elimination of filariasis, as follows: after basic elimination of filariasis for ten years or more at the county-level, and achieving (i) etiological monitoring, covering more than 3% of the resident population, no positive microfilariae; and (ii) mosquito vector monitoring, no human filarial larva found in mosquitoes.[16]

Diagnosis

Filariasis is usually diagnosed by identifying microfilariae on a Giemsa-stained thick blood film, using the "gold standard" known as the finger prick test. The finger prick test draws blood from the capillaries of the fingertip; larger veins can be used for blood extraction, however, strict time of day windows must be observed. Blood must be drawn at appropriate times, reflecting the feeding activities of the vector. For example, for *W. bancrofti*, the vector of which is a mosquito, the night is the preferred time for blood collection. *Loa loa*'s vector is the deer fly, and so, daytime collection is preferred. This method of diagnosis is only appropriate for microfilariae that use blood as the transport from the lungs to the skin. Some filarial worms, such as *Mansonella streptocerca* and *Onchocerca volvulus*, produce microfilariae that do not use the blood; they reside in the skin only. For these worms, diagnosis relies upon skin snips and can be carried out at any time.

Various concentration methods can be applied such as the membrane filter, Knott's concentration method, and sedimentation technique.

Polymerase chain reaction and antigenic assays, which detect circulating filarial antigens, are also available for diagnosis. The latter are particularly useful in amicrofilaremic cases. Spot tests for antigen are far more sensitive, and allow the test to be done at any time.[17]

Lymph node aspirate and chylus fluid may also yield microfilariae. Medical imaging, such as CT or MRI, may reveal a "filarial dance sign" in chylus fluid; X-rays can show calcified adult worms in lymphatics. The DEC provocation test is performed to obtain satisfying numbers of parasites in daytime samples. Xenodiagnosis is now obsolete, and eosinophilia is a nonspecific primary sign.[18]

Treatment

- Hetrazan can kill both *W. bancrofti* and *B. malayi*. It has better effect on killing microfilariae than adult worms; it may cause mild adverse events such as fever, headache, and nausea, etc. The dosage is 300 mg twice per day, with continuous treating for 7 days.
- Furapyrimidone also can kill both *W. bancrofti* and *B. malayi*. It has better effect on killing adult worms than microfilariae. The dosage is 10 mg/kg, twice per day, with continuous treating for 7 days.

References

1. Ravindran B. Filariasis control: ethics, economics, and good science. Lancet, 2001, 358(9277): 246.

2. Spencer J, Owen-Smith M. Filariasis. Lancet, 1966, 1(7434): 427-428.

3. Control of filariasis. Lancet, 1952, 2(6740): 872.

4. Shi FT, Ling XM, Shi HH, et al. Assessment of intracutaneous test in longitudinal surveillance for lymphatic filariasis. Zhongguo Ji Sheng Chong Xue Yu Ji Sheng Chong Bing Za Zhi, 1989, 7(4): 280-283. (In Chinese)

5. Pan SX, Xie ZY, Lu XG, et al. On the transmission role of residual microfilaremia cases in the area with filariasis virtually eradicated. Zhongguo Ji Sheng Chong Xue Yu Ji Sheng Chong Bing Za Zhi, 1990, 8(3): 191-194. (In Chinese)

6. Xu L, Jiang Z, Yu S, et al. Nationwide survey of the distribution of human parasites in China--infection with parasite species in human population. Zhongguo Ji Sheng Chong Xue Yu Ji Sheng Chong Bing Za Zhi, 1995, 13(1): 1-7. (In Chinese)

7. Ndeffo-Mbah ML, Galvani AP. Global elimination of lymphatic filariasis. Lancet Infect Dis, 2017, 17(4): 358-359.

8. Shi Z, Sun D. Achievements in the research on filariasis in China in the past 50 years. Zhongguo Ji Sheng Chong Xue Yu Ji Sheng Chong Bing Za Zhi, 1999, 17(5): 267-270. (In Chinese)

9. Cao NX, Xue MJ, Li GH, et al. Surveillance of schistosomiasis, malaria and filariasis in the

mobile population in Jiashan County, 1989–2000. Zhongguo Ji Sheng Chong Xue Yu Ji Sheng Chong Bing Za Zhi, 2004, 22(3): 188. (In Chinese)

10. Zhou YZ, Sun DJ, Liu W. Preliminary establishment of data-managing information system of filariasis. Zhongguo Ji Sheng Chong Xue Yu Ji Sheng Chong Bing Za Zhi, 2000, 18(1): 60-61. (In Chinese)

11. Sun DJ. Global significance of the elimination of lymphatic filariasis in China. Zhongguo Ji Sheng Chong Xue Yu Ji Sheng Chong Bing Za Zhi, 2005, 23(5 Suppl): 329-331. (In Chinese)

12. Pan SX, Lu XG, Xie ZY, et al. Long-term surveillance after basic elimination of bancroftian filariasis. Zhongguo Ji Sheng Chong Xue Yu Ji Sheng Chong Bing Za Zhi, 1993, 11(1): 21-24. (In Chinese)

13. Li TD. Views on a non-endemic area for filariasis in Yunan Province. Zhongguo Ji Sheng Chong Xue Yu Ji Sheng Chong Bing Za Zhi, 2000, 18(4): 196. (In Chinese)

14. Zhan FX, Zhang S Q, Wang LL, et al. Lymphatic filariasis in Hubei Province: from prevailing to elimination. Zhongguo Ji Sheng Chong Xue Yu Ji Sheng Chong Bing Za Zhi, 2012, 30(1): 65-70. (In Chinese)

15. Yang JM, Kang YM, Zhang WQ, et al. Study on strategy of filariasis control in Heze City. Zhongguo Ji Sheng Chong Xue Yu Ji Sheng Chong Bing Za Zhi, 2005, 23(5): 318-319. (In Chinese)

16. Li ZH, Zhang KZ, Yan YF. Evaluation on surveillance and intervention of lymphatic filariasis after interruption of the disease transmission in Jiangxi province. Zhongguo Ji Sheng Chong Xue Yu Ji Sheng Chong Bing Za Zhi, 2002, 20(4): 249-250. (In Chinese)

17. Duan J, Li Q, Li Z, et al. SurveilLance on filariasis after its basic elimination in Hunan Province. Zhongguo Ji Sheng Chong Xue Yu Ji Sheng Chong Bing Za Zhi, 1998, 16(4): 291-295. (In Chinese)

18. Cheng XZ, Kong DY, Li ZC. Filariasis elimination in Zoucheng City of Shandong Province: measures and effect. Zhongguo Ji Sheng Chong Xue Yu Ji Sheng Chong Bing Za Zhi, 2006, 24(1): 3-6. (In Chinese)

1.3.2　Visceral leishmaniasis

Leishmaniasis, a zoonotic disease caused by *Leishmania*, is transmitted between arthropods and mammals. The disease is reported in more than 80 countries, with an estimated 15 million patients and more than 400,000 new cases each year in the world before the new century. *Leishmania* may be a conditionally pathogenic parasite for human immunodeficiency virus (HIV)-infected individuals.

Leishmaniasis is a protozoal disease caused by *Leishmania* parasites in human and animal cells. Visceral leishmaniasis (VL), or kala-azar, causes parasitism in visceral macrophages and visceral lesions. Cutaneous leishmaniasis causes skin lesions in macrophages that parasitize the skin; it is also called the "Oriental sore".[1]

The prevalence of VL in China is very widespread, affecting 17 provinces and cities. According to a 1951 survey, an estimated 530,000 patients had VL, with a large number of infected dogs.[4] At that time, leishmaniasis was very popular in plain areas such as northern Jiangsu, northern Anhui, southern Shandong, eastern Henan, southern Hebei, northern suburbs of Hubei, northeastern Hubei, and Shanxi. Among them, Shandong is the area where the VL epidemic is the most serious. Meanwhile, leishmaniasis in hilly and mountainous areas are moderate, such as the northwestern suburbs of Gansu, Ningxia, Qinghai, northern Shaanxi, western Henan, Shanxi, northern Hebei, Liaoning, and Beijing. [2]

Epidemiology

According to the prevalence relating to different geographical features and sources of infection, there are three types of VL, namely plains or human type, hill or zoonotic type, and desert or wild animal source type. Due to its vast territory and wide range of diseases, all the three types exist in China.[3]

Type 1: Plains or anthroponotic type. Occurring in plains areas, local VL spreads mainly among humans, and infected humans are sources of infection. The incidence of the disease in humans is high, and there may be a pandemic. Patients are predominately older children and youth, while infants are less affected. This type of VL is not very common in dogs; *Phlebotomus chinensis* is the vector that transmits the disease to dogs. The use of integrated measures such as treatment of patients and elimination of the vectors generally allows the incidence to be brought under control.

Type 2: Hill or animal zoonotic type. This type exists in the hills area and the Loess Plateau such as northwestern suburbs of Gansu, Ningxia, Qinghai, northern Shaanxi, western Henan, Shanxi, northern Hebei, Liaoning, and Beijing, with the infection rate higher in dogs than in humans. Infected dogs are a direct source of infection of human VL. Normally, patients lived separately, and the association between patients is not obvious. Patients are predominately young children aged less than 10 years, and infant morbidity is also high. In this type, *P. chinensis* has a wild living habitat, thus the decontamination method of stagnant spray effect is insignificant. Wild animals in areas with this type of VL are likely to be reservoir hosts.

Type 3: Desert or wildlife source type. Also known as natural foci, this type is a disease of wild animals that spontaneously spreads among animals independently of human existence and thus becomes a natural source of VL. It is distributed in desert and semi-desert areas of northwest China. Humans have been infected during the course of reclamation in wasteland or other activities, and the disease is transmitted from wild animals to people by sand flies. Patients are widely scattered, and most are children aged less than three years; this type affects very few adult patients. The infection can sometimes be manifested as lymph node kala-azar. The vectors are wild *Phlebotomus wui* and *Phlebotomus alexandri*. In areas with this type of VL, it is extremely easy to observe a natural infection through sandfly.

In China, the first case report of VL was in 1880 in Jining, Shandong Province, and it was confirmed that there was VL in other counties of this province. In 1912, a patient in Henan Province was confirmed infected with *Leishmania*, by liver puncture. Since then, VL cases have been continuously reported in Henan. By 1923, VL had spread to 36 counties. In 1923, according to an analysis of 171 VL cases treated at the Anhui Minzhi Hospital, 14 counties in Anhui were identified as endemic areas for VL. The contagious character of the disease itself and, as it was found to be incurable early on, led to the spread of VL, which not only occurred year after year but intensified with time. Overall, the trend was that prevalence was increasing and a rising trend was observed in the total number of patients. After the 1931 floods in the Yangtze and Huaihe Rivers, the prevalence of the disease increased day by day, with a marked increase in the number of infected people every year. The impact of the disease burden on China became increasingly heavy and showed signs of widespread sprawl. At that time, eight provinces had the highest number of VL cases, including Shandong, Hebei, Anhui, Jiangsu, Henan, Gansu, Shaanxi, and Liaoning.

Sand flies are the intermediate host of VL. Their larvae will hide in environments of suitable temperature and humidity for overwintering. This environment is loose soil and places containing organic matter, such as corners of the house, barns, toilets, caves, wall seams, cellars, bridge holes, etc. Between 1910 and 1949, most of the residential areas in China had grass and soil walls that were not whitewashed, with many gaps, making them an excellent place for the larvae to thrive. In addition, the awareness of the public was weak: people had toilets very close to housing, garbage was everywhere, etc. Summer is the perfect season for infection, with sandflies fluttering and people barely wanting to sleep during the nights, leading to sand flies easily biting them. Both the natural environment and living environment are ideal places for sand flies to breed. Due to this, the increasing epidemic trend for VL was unstoppable at that time. The epidemic situation in rural areas was much worse than in urban areas.

There were two main reasons that explained the serious prevalence of VL in the rural areas of China during that time. The first was the poor economy. People wore rags and did not have enough food. Most were living in shabby huts, with several people sleeping on one bed. People had very poor physical fitness and could become easily infected with many diseases. They also had no money for treatment, resulting in the course of VL being very long and the disease spreading easily. At that time, neostibosan, a special medicine imported from Germany, could cure VL. However, the drug was costly and needed long-term injections, with one patient requiring one year's worth of living expenses to be cured. The other reason was the poor living conditions (dirty food and clothing; high humidity bedrooms; house mixed with kitchen, livestock, and poultry; and pests, flies, and mosquitoes everywhere) and weak public health awareness. As intermediate hosts of VL, sand flies prefer to live in animal stables that are damp and dark and characterized by air boring. The living environment in rural areas provides a suitable environment for breeding of sandflies. Compared with rural areas, there are fewer domestic animals in cities, and no place for breeding livestock, thereby, there are fewer or even no sand flies. However, patients who come to and from the city for medical treatment during the day are less likely to enhance the transmission pattern.

Control strategy

After the People's Republic of China was founded, the prevalence of kala-azar was also very widespread, affecting 17 provinces and cities. According to a survey in 1951, there were an estimated 530,000 patients in various provinces, as described in section 1.3.3.

In 1951, the Ministry of Health of China declared VL as an infectious disease that urgently needed to be eliminated. At that time, the vast north rural areas of the Yangtze River, comprising 16 provinces, municipalities, and autonomous regions, were highly endemic for VL. Shandong, Jiangsu, Anhui, Henan, and Hebei were severely endemic areas, followed by Shanxi, Gansu, and Xinjiang, while the other provinces were only mildly endemic. After active prevention and control, VL was basically eliminated in 1958. However, since the 1990s, there has been a resurgence of VL in China. Recently (from 2008 to 2018), six western provinces (Xinjiang, Gansu, Inner Mongolia, Shaanxi, Shanxi, and Sichuan) have reported sporadic cases.

In VL endemic areas, the local government and relevant departments have taken measures such as eliminating dogs, washing dogs with pesticides, and sand flies control with nets, to monitoring the spread of VL. The implementation of these measures focused on eliminating the infectious source and the sand fly, and blocking the sand fly interactions between dogs and dogs, and between dogs and people, with remarkable results achieved. In addition, on the basis of consolidating the achievements made in prevention and treatment, a monitoring system has been established. In areas where the epidemic of VL has been controlled, the distribution and density of sand fly is regularly monitored to prevent a resurgence. This is done by joining forces in a planned way, thoroughly investigating and determining the distribution of pathogens and vectors, and adopting decisive measures to control the epidemic. For example, in 1991 and 1993, Li County, Sichuan Province adopted a total ban on dogs in affected areas and banned domestic dogs for three and five years, respectively. The number of VL cases has decreased significantly since 1994. In addition, since 2002, many local governments have started creating a file on VL unique to every infected person. It includes names, ages, addresses, dates of onset, and other items relating to infected persons. It also includes detailed records of each patient's diagnosis, treatment, etc. In addition, health education activities aimed at residents living in VL endemic areas have significantly raised the awareness of local residents in disease prevention and control, and laid down a good foundation for the control of VL.

Although the VL prevention and control measures adopted for different epidemics and prevalence ranges have minimized the harm to the population, none have completely eradicated the source of infection. For example, dogs are commonly used for guarding houses, orchards, and crops, and therefore there is a great resistance to dog killing. In addition, transfer of cases, hiding of dogs, and conflict with dog killing have come up. At present, the number of domestic dogs in endemic areas is gradually increasing. If there is a source of infection or imported source of infection in the area, VL is likely to occur again. In addition, the vector is widely distributed in prevailing areas of barren hills, and controlling and eliminating wildlife alone is difficult to do. Wild animal hosts are likely to pass *Leishmania* spp. on to domestic animals and humans through sand flies. Epidemiological surveys show that infection of individuals in recent years appears to be related to their direct entry into the wilderness. However, changing the habitat can effectively destroy the breeding and habitat of certain species tied to VL transmission becoming extinct. The challenge that appears now to the centers for diseases control and prevention, is how people could be protected from the attack of naturally occurring epidemics if natural habitats are preserved.

Diagnosis

VL is diagnosed by either demonstration of amastigotes (Leishman-Donovan [LD] bodies, aflagellar forms) in splenic or bone marrow smears or by culture of *Leishmania* promastigotes (flagellar forms) from a clinical specimen (most commonly in NNN media). While the sensitivity of splenic smears could be as high as >95%, they carry the risk of severe/fatal hemorrhage. Bone marrow aspiration is painful, cumbersome, and has a low sensitivity (60–85%). Culture cannot be used for routine clinical diagnosis as it requires expensive equipment and expertise. In addition to the difficulties associated with splenic aspiration, technical expertise remains a necessity for proper staining and microscopic demonstration of parasites.

As for various other diseases, specific serodiagnostics for antibody detection have been employed in VL diagnosis. Conventional methods for antibody detection include gel diffusion, complement fixation (CF) test, indirect hemagglutination assay (IHA), immunofluorescent assay (IFA), and countercurrent immunoelectrophoresis.

However these tests are limited not only by practical challenges at peripheral laboratories, as they require adequate facilities and expertise, but also their sensitivities and specificities are not high, as antigens may have cross-reactivity with sera from patients with other infections. The direct agglutination (DA) test, based on the agglutination of trypsinized whole promastigotes, has been found to be useful in several endemic countries. Various studies, including from India, have shown that DA tests are 91–100% of sensitivity and 72–100% of specificity.

ELISA has been used as a serodiagnostic tool in leishmaniasis diagnosis. The technique is highly sensitive, but its specificity depends on the antigen used. Several antigens have been tried. The most common one is a crude soluble antigen (CSA) derived by lysing the *Leishmania* promastigotes. Its sensitivity is about 80–100%, but cross-reactions with sera from patients of malaria, tuberculosis, and toxoplasmosis have been recorded. An amastigote-specific recombinant 39 amino acid antigen (rK39) derived from *L. chagasi* (etiological organism for kala-azar in Brazil), has been shown to be specific for antibodies in patients with VL caused by members of the *L. donovani* complex. This antigen, encoded by 117 base pairs of genes conserved in the kinesin region of the parasite, is highly sensitive and predictive of the disease.

In Indian VL, anti-rK39 antibody titers were 59-fold higher than those of antibodies against CSA at the time of diagnosis, falling sharply with successful therapy during post-treatment and follow-up periods. The widespread application of these techniques, of which some are excellent, has been prevented by the need for sophisticated equipment, skilled human resources, electricity, and because of their high cost.[4]

Due to the difficult conditions in areas of endemicity, there has been an urgent need for a simple, cheap, rapid, and accurate test with a high sensitivity and specificity to be developed. A promising ready-to-use immunochromatographic strip test based on the rk39 antigen has been developed as a rapid test for use in difficult field conditions. In their study, Goswami et al. reported on the successful use of this rapid test in the diagnosis of kala-azar in West Bengal. In the Indian subcontinent, this rapid strip test has been very successful, though not so much in Europe or Africa.

Notwithstanding these limitations, the rK39 immunochromatographic strip test has proven to be versatile in predicting acute infection. It is the only available method for diagnosing VL with acceptable sensitivity and specificity levels, and is also simple and inexpensive (US$ 1 to 1.5 for each strip). It can yield a positive result very early in the course of the disease.[5] Recently, the Food and Drug Administration of the United States (US FDA) has approved the rK39 strip test from InBios International, USA, for VL diagnosis. Another format of this test by DiaMed, Switzerland is under evaluation.

Another diagnostic method is antigen detection, which is more specific than antibody-based techniques. This method is also useful to diagnose the disease in cases where there is deficient antibody production (as in acquired immune deficiency (AIDS) patients). A new latex agglutination (LA) test, KAtex, using monoclonal antibodies for detecting leishmanial antigen in urine of patients with VL has shown sensitivities between 68% and 100%, and a specificity of 100% in preliminary trials. The antigen is detected quite early during the infection, and the results of animal experiments suggest that the amount of detectable antigen tends to decline rapidly following chemotherapy. These antigens are also detectable in blood and efforts are underway towards further refining this test.

Detection of parasitic DNA in the blood after polymerase chain reaction (PCR) amplification has also been applied in the clinical diagnosis of VL, and several Indian laboratories have developed primers that are species-specific and are able to detect very low levels of parasitemia. However, the technique is yet to be standardized for clinical application in India. Polymerase chain reaction has the potential to predict cure or detect early relapse. However, as it is highly sophisticated, it needs expensive equipment, skilled personnel, and the running cost is likely to be very high. In a study reported from India, the sensitivity of PCR with whole blood was 96% and 93.8% for VL and post-VL dermal leishmaniasis, respectively.

Parasite diagnosis by splenic and marrow smear examination remains the "gold standard", with its usual limitations. The rK39 strip test is an important step forward in the diagnosis of VL, and it has the potential to be used under field conditions. The rK39-based diagnostic has already become popular in other tests, which are likely candidates for the diagnosis and prognosis of leishmaniasis in the future, such as KAtex and a field-adaptable version of PCR, which has to be simple, inexpensive, and easily available.[6]

Treatment

Sodium stibogluconate

Six days treatment: Total dosage of 100 mg/kg for adults or total dosage of 150–170 mg/kg for children, in six days, through intramuscular injection or intravenous injection.

Three weeks treatment: Usually for serious infection. Total dosage of 150 mg/kg for adults or total dosage of 200 mg/kg for children, in three weeks, through intramuscular injection or intravenous injection.

References

1. Moore TA. Visceral leishmaniasis. N Engl J Med, 1997, 336: 965.

2. Zhong HL, Zhang NZ. Studies on leishmaniasis in China. Historical background, epidemiology, clinical aspects, legislature and control program. Chin Med J (Engl), 1986, 99: 281-300.

3. Lun ZR, Wu MS, Chen YF, et al. Visceral Leishmaniasis in China: an Endemic Disease under Control. Clin Microbiol Rev, 2015, 28: 987-1004.

4. Bangert M, Flores-Chavez MD, Llanes-Acevedo IP, et al. Validation of rK39 immunochromatographic test and direct agglutination test for the diagnosis of Mediterranean visceral leishmaniasis in Spain. PLoS Negl Trop Dis, 2018, 12: e6277.

5. Maia Z, Lirio M, Mistro S, Mendes CM, et al. Comparative study of rK39 Leishmania antigen for serodiagnosis of visceral leishmaniasis: systematic review with meta-analysis. PLoS Negl Trop Dis, 2012, 6: e1484.

6. Sakkas H, Gartzonika C, Levidiotou S. Laboratory diagnosis of human visceral leishmaniasis. J Vector Borne Dis, 2016, 53: 8-16.

1.3.3 Human babesiosis

Human babesiosis is an emerging tick-borne parasitic disease caused by the protozoa of the genus *Babesia*, a kind of blood-feeding parasite. *Babesia* spp. has long been considered as a pathogen of domesticated and wild animals. In the last 50 years, *Babesia* spp. has increasingly been identified as a cause of infection in humans worldwide.

The first human babesiosis case was reported in 1957 near Zagreb, Croatia. A farmer pastured cattle on tick-infested grazing, and then presented with fever, anemia, and hemoglobinuria. He was asplenic and died of renal insufficiency during the second week of illness. The causative agent was most likely *Babesia divergens*, but was initially reported as *B. bovis*. In 1968, another case caused by *B. divergens* was confirmed in an asplenic patient in Ireland. Meanwhile, several cases of human babesiosis were diagnosed in Nantucket Island, Massachusetts, USA. The pathogen was identified as *B. microti*, which usually infects small rodents (e.g. mice). Subsequently, *Ixodes dammini* and the white-tailed deer (*Odocoileus virginianus*) were identified as a vector and an important natural host, respectively. In the 1990s, *B. duncani* (WA1) was identified in human cases reported from the northern Pacific coast. Another *Babesia* spp. (EU1), closely related to *B. odocoilei*, was identified in 2003 in patients from Austria and Italy. Another two species pathogenic to humans, KO1 and TW1, have been identified in Korea, and Taiwan of China, respectively.

Epidemiology

The life cycles of *Babesia* parasites are not yet fully clear. The only confirmed vectors of *Babesia* spp. are from the Ixodidae family. The life cycle of *I. scapularis* and its role in *B. microti* transmission has been well documented. *Ixodes scapularis* is prevalent in eastern USA and Canada. Briefly, the larva and nymph stages both suck blood from their rodent hosts for maturity. It is estimated that up to 60% of the rodents are infected with *B. microti*. Then, the adult ticks feed on deer as a permanent food source. Newly hatched larval stages take a blood meal from their vertebrate host at the end of summer. During winter, when they are dormant and molt into nymph stages, the parasites cross the tick gut epithelium and travel to the salivary glands. It has been shown that these parasites require some activation from exposure to warm-blooded hosts to generate active sporozoites once the ticks feed again. The following summer, the nymph stages are required to feed again in preparation for development into adults later that year; they are now able to transmit parasites into the vertebrate host. It is at this stage of tick development that zoonotic infection into the human host occurs. The adult stages of *I. scapularis* feed primarily on *O. virginianus*, which are not reservoirs for *B. microti*, but may be a direct contributor to the expansion of *Ixodes* ticks and babesiosis in general. *Babesia divergens* is transmitted by the *I. ricinus* tick, whose life cycle lasts for three years, as the larvae, nymphs, and adults each mature in consecutive years. Most tick-borne infections are reported between April and October, which coincides not only with the warmer weather in the northern hemisphere when ticks are more active, but also when individuals spend more time in tick-infested areas.

When *Babesia* spp. sporozoites are first injected into the human host, they target the host's red blood cells (RBCs) immediately, unlike *Plasmodium* spp., which are required to undergo an exoerythrocytic phase in the hepatic cells. Furthermore, infected RBCs remain circulating in the peripheral blood stream, including regularly passing through the host's spleen, and do not sequester to the fine capillaries of the bone marrow or organs. It is the parasite's ability to first recognize and then invade the host's RBCs that is central to human babesiosis; the parasites invade RBCs using multiple complex interactions between parasite proteins and the host cell surface, which are not yet fully elucidated. Once inside the RBCs, the parasite begins a cycle of maturation and growth. The early stages of the cycle are morphologically indistinguishable from *Plasmodium* spp., with both appearing as ring-like parasites. Replication occurs by budding, where one ring form divides into two, often referred to as the "figure eight" form. Budding may occur again, giving rise to the tetrad form known as a "Maltese cross". Both these morphological forms are unique to *Babesia* spp. and are the basis of definitive diagnosis by microscopy, especially if *Plasmodium* spp. are also suspected. Once the parasites have concluded division, the resulting merozoites egress from the RBCs, destroying them in the process and seeking new, uninfected RBCs to invade, perpetuating the intracellular cycle of infection.

Emerging Babesia species infections in China

Since 1982, eleven *Babesia* species have been reported in mainland China: *B. orientalis*, *B. ovis*, *B. major*, *B. ovata*, *B. caballi*, *B. motasi*, *Babesia* sp. Kashi, *B. microti*, *Babesia* sp. Xinjiang, *B. divergens*, and *B. venatorum*. Among them, three species (*B. divergens*, *B. microti*, and *B. venatorum*) are pathogenic to humans.

Tick and animal infections

There are several babesiosis natural foci areas in China. Surveys conducted in Heilongjiang, Jilin, Xinjiang Uygur Autonomous Region, Fujian, Inner Mongolia Autonomous Region, Zhejiang, Taiwan, Guangxi Zhuang Autonomous Region, and Henan confirmed the presence of *Babesia* in ticks and/or other reservoir hosts. The above areas are natural foci of piroplasms and represent a hazard to public health.

Babesia microti was confirmed in dogs and in *Haemaphysalis longicornis* ticks in Henan; in rodents in Zhejiang, Fujian, Heilongjiang, and Henan; and in *H. concinna* and *I. persulcatus* ticks, reed voles (*Microtus fortis*), and striped field mice in Heilongjiang. *Babesia divergens* was identified in *I. persulcatus*, *H. japonica*, and *H. concinna* ticks and striped field mice in many areas of Heilongjiang. In forested areas of northeastern China, *B. venatorum* was detected in *I. persulcatus* ticks.

Ixodes persulcatus is considered as the most important vector for the transmission of human tick-borne diseases in China. In addition, there is anecdotal evidence that *I. persulcatus* ticks can transmit *B. microti* and *B. divergens* to both humans and animals. The results of a survey conducted in Heilongjiang revealed that 78% of all the *Babesia* infections in *I. persulcatus* were caused by *B. microti*, while the remaining cases were infected with *B. divergens*. Among *H. concinna* species, the second most important tick, 82% of the cases were infected with *B. microti* and the remaining with *B. divergens*. Another molecular survey conducted in Jilin showed that *B. microti* was the main pathogenic strain in *I. persulcatus* with an infection rate of 5%, suggesting that *B. microti* may be the dominant species in northeastern China. Moreover, a molecular survey conducted in the Inner Mongolia Autonomous Region revealed that *Dermacentor nuttalli* was the predominant tick species, with 66% (29/44) infected with *B. divergens* and 34% (15/44) with *B. microti*.

In summary, epidemiological studies have demonstrated the wide occurrence of pathogenic *Babesia* spp. in China. Specific PCR especially has demonstrated that *B. microti* was the dominant species in northeastern and southeastern China; *B. divergens* and other *Babesia* species may be the main pathogen species in Xinjiang Uygur Autonomous Region and Inner Mongolia.

Human infections

Babesia microti, *B. divergens*, and *B. venatorum* have been reported to infect humans in mainland China. *Babesia* are intra-erythrocytic protozoans and show similar symptoms of inflammation when compared with *Plasmodium* species in clinical manifestations, including headaches, myalgia, fever, vomiting, chills, anemia with hypotension, nausea, altered mental status, respiratory distress, hepatomegaly, and renal insufficiency.

From 1931 to 1944, Hung reported on a series of cases of human parasitemia in Beibei, Chongqing. Protozoa were observed in human erythrocytes, which showed similar characteristics to the ring stage of *Plasmodium falciparum*. However, the parasites were obviously smaller and no pigment was presented, thus strongly indicating that they were *Babesia*. In 2009, two cases of *B. divergens* infection were confirmed among 377 patients with anemia in Shandong. In 2011, by using bone marrow and peripheral blood smears and PCR analysis, a patient was diagnosed with *B. microti* infection in Zhejiang. Between 2012 and 2013, utilizing PCR, 10 cases among 449 febrile patients with malaria-like symptoms were confirmed with *B. microti* infection in Yunnan. From 1984 to 2014, of all reported human cases in China, 16 cases were confirmed with *Babesia* species infection, among which 14 cases were infected with *B. microti* and two with *B. divergens*. Over half of the above cases were originally infected in south or southeast China (Table 1.5). Particularly, 48 cases of *B. venatorum* infections were reported at a sentinel hospital in northeastern China between 2011 and 2014. Among them, 32 cases were confirmed, and the remaining were probable. It is noteworthy that this was the first report of endemic human *B. venatorum* infections anywhere worldwide. In addition, two cases infected with uncharacterized *Babesia* species were reported in Yunnan in southwestern China in 1982 and 2008 (see Table 1.5).

Diagnosis

Direct detection

The microscopic examination of *Babesia* parasites with Wright's- or Giemsa-stained blood smears is the classic diagnostic method. However, its limitation is that it is difficult to directly examine parasites in less than 0.1–0.5% parasitemia. Thus, it is not recommended for diagnosis in some chronic and asymptomatic cases. As parasitemia of more than 5% is rarely seen in mild cases, serial films are still highly recommended.

The intracellular trophozoites and extracellular merozoites are usually oval or ring shaped, with a red or pink chromatin and a blue or purple cytoplasm (Figure 1.2).

Table 1.5   Clinical and laboratory findings of humans infected with emerging
tick-borne *Babesia* in mainland China.

	Humans infected with…			
	B. divergens (*N* = 2)	*B. microti* (*N* = 11)	*B. venatorum* (*N* = 49)	Uncharacterized (*N* = 3)
Male/total	2/2	6/11	19/49	0/1
Age range (years)	47, 55	8–48	1–75	
Clinical manifestation				
Fever	2/2	11/11	22/49	1/1
Malaise	–	1/1	1/1	1/1
Myalgia	–	1/1	6/49	3/3
Fatigue	2/2	1/1	15/49	3/3
Anemia	–	1/1	8/49	2/2
Weakness	–	1/2	1/1	1/1
Chills	–	11/11	3/48	1/1
Shortness of breath	–	1/1	1/1	–
Cough	–	1/1	–	–
Anorexia	–	1/1	–	2/2
Weight loss	–	1/1	–	–
Dizziness	–	1/1	8/48	–
Headache	–	1/1	13/48	–
Arthralgia	–	1/1	7/48	1/1
Laboratory test*				
Leukopenia	2/2	0/1	3/48	–
Thrombocytopenia	2/2	0/1	5/49	–
Elevated alanine aminotransferase	2/2	1/1	7/14	–
Elevated aspartate aminotransferase	2/2	1/1	7/14	–
Elevated lactate dehydrogenase	2/2	–	1/1	–
Elevated leukocyte count	–	–	1/1	–
Elevated C-reactive protein	2/2	–	5/8	–
Elevated procalcitonin	–	–	1/1	–
Elevated total bilirubin	–	–	2/7	–
Hepatic injury	2/2	1/1	–	–
Hemoglobinuria	2/2	1/1	–	–
Renal failure	2/2	1/1	–	–

–, indicates that data were not reported or the test was not performed, or the data could not be extracted from literature.

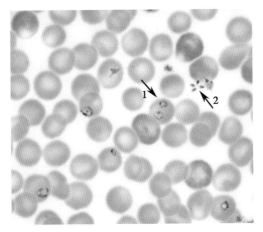

Figure 1.2   Standard asynchronous in vitro culture of
B. divergens in RBCs with a classic morphological ring
(1) and Maltese cross (2) forms.

In terms of species identification, generally it is impossible to distinguish *Babesia* spp. from each other morphologically, as this requires more sensitive detection methods based on PCR. Moreover, it is very difficult to tell the difference between the early ring stages of *Babesia* spp. and some blood stages of *Plasmodium* spp., with the differential diagnosis being the observation of the tetrad or "Maltese cross" forms.

The PCR diagnostic assay, particularly real-time or quantitative PCR, shows much more sensitivity than microscopy, and is becoming a common technique for the detection of *B. microti*. Furthermore, the extensive use of PCR technology makes high-throughput screening more and applicable.

Indirect detection

As *Babesia* parasites cannot always be observed in chronic infections, serological testing, usually immunofluorescence assay, could be utilized to support clinical diagnostics of human babesiosis. Nearly all asymptomatic chronic *B. microti* infections seroconvert in immunocompetent individuals, but the presence of anti-*B. microti* antibodies merely suggests an infection at some point in time, as *B. microti*-specific IgG titers of 1:64 have been detected for up 12 months after the parasite infection has cleared. Immunoglobulin G (IgG) titers over 1:1024, however, exhibit good correlation with acute *B. microti* infection, and serve as an accurate indicator of recent infection and the occurrence of *Babesia*-specific IgM. However, in severe cases (e.g.

B. divergens-infected or immunocompromised individuals), direct detection methods rather than serology are usually suitable for diagnosis, as there is an urgent need for treatment to prevent the host from generating anti-*Babesia* antibodies.

Treatment

In 1982, the combination of quinine and clindamycin was first applied for babesiosis treatment in a newborn infant. Subsequently, this has become the choice of treatment for babesiosis. In most cases, this treatment is effective to clear the infection, with treatment failures reported in patients with splenectomy or HIV infection. Furthermore, this combined treatment can supervene side effects such as tinnitus, vertigo, and gastrointestinal upset.

The combination of azithromycin and atovaquone is a useful alternative for human babesiosis treatment, and generally achieves better results than the combination of quinine and clindamycin. The combination of azithromycin (500 mg on day 1, 250 mg/day thereafter) and atovaquone (750 mg every 12 hours) is as effective as the combination of quinine (650 mg every eight hours) and clindamycin (600 mg every six hours) in clearing parasitemia and resolving symptoms. The recommended therapy for babesiosis is summarized in Table 1.6.

Table 1.6 Recommended therapies to treat babesiosis.

Antibiotic[a]	Dose	Frequency
Clindamycin	Adult: 600 mg Child: 5–10 mg/kg	Every 6 hours
and		
Quinine	Adult: 650 mg Child: 8.3 mg/kg	Every 8 hours
OR		
Atovaquone	Adult: 750 mg Child: 20 mg/kg	Every 12 hours
and		
Azithromycin	Adult: 500–600 mg 250–600 mg Child: 12 mg/kg	On day 1 On subsequent days

[a]All antibiotics are administered for 7–10 days.

Exchange transfusion is considered as a potentially lifesaving therapy for patients suffering from severe infections, especially those with high parasitemia (more than 5%), significant hemolysis, or pulmonary or renal compromise. Either partial or full blood volume exchange transfusion may be applied depending on the severity of the disease. This procedure should only be used for severe babesiosis cases due to the associated risks of blood exposure.

Drug resistance

Generally, the two main treatment options remain effective, but problems with the onset time of drugs and parasite persistence have been found both in Europe[1] and USA[2]. Although drug resistance is not suspected in these cases, patient parasitemia should be monitored throughout treatment. However, three incidents of drug resistance to azithromycin and atovaquone were reported in immunocompromised patients infected with *B. microti* in USA, which was defined by relapse 28 days after treatment.[3] Given the lack of alternative chemotherapeutics, there is a pressing need for new chemical entities to be discovered for babesiosis treatment.

Current challenges

Due to the low level parasitemia of babesiosis in the early stage of the disease course, it is strongly suggested that at least 300 microscopic fields should be reviewed before obtaining diagnostic results, which limits the application of microscopy in the field. On the other hand, a specific PCR test could identify the *Babesia* spp. and distinguish it from *Plasmodium* infections. It is, however, relatively difficult to perform molecular methodology in field surveys due to the high cost and skill requirement.

Major problems around the diagnosis of *Babesia* infections are attributed to the general lack of clinical awareness of babesiosis in the medical community, the nonspecific clinical manifestations, and the absence of simple and effective rapid diagnostic tests (RDTs). Rapid diagnostic tests for human babesiosis have not been established and are not yet readily available at almost all of the routine diagnostic laboratories. Furthermore, conventional laboratory test results in human babesiosis patients may be nonspecific and misleading, including high levels of transaminases, alkaline unconjugated bilirubin, phosphatases, lactic dehydrogenase, normochromia, normocytic anemia, and thrombocytopenia.

Referring to the immunological diagnosis of babesiosis, the IFA is considered the standard assay for detecting the *Babesia* antibody. Immunoblot assay for antibody detection is another option. A novel *B. microti* secreted antigen (BmSA1) identified by Luo et al.[4] could serve as a universal and promising target for the serodiagnosis of human babesiosis. Ooka and colleagues[5] performed an ELISA for the diagnosis of *B. microti* infection using rBmP94/CT, which exhibited a high sensitivity and specificity in mice infected with *B. microti* and other species of *Babesia*. These results demonstrate that rBmP94/CT and BmSA1 could be used as promising markers for human babesiosis surveillance. In New England in USA, an immunofluorescence assay has been performed to evaluate acute babesiosis cases. The sensitivity and specificity were 91% and 99%, respectively, which revealed that the assay could be used as a sensitive and specific clinical diagnostic method for babesiosis.

A survey on seroprevalence of blood donors was conducted in the Upper Midwest and Northeast US, which are *Babesia* endemic areas. Indirect immunofluorescence assay was applied to detect the *B. microti* infection. It showed that almost 2% (42/2,150) of the donors tested positive and, especially, one patient was confirmed to contract an ongoing *Babesia* infection by positive PCR results (1/42).[6] However, most of the seropositive cases (41/42) tested negative in the molecular survey. Thus, clinical diagnosis of human babesiosis can be further complicated by persistent low parasitemia or asymptomatic latent infections, particularly in malaria and babesiosis syndemic areas.

References

1. Haselbarth K, Tenter AM, Brade V, et al. First case of human babesiosis in Germany - Clinical presentation and molecular characterisation of the pathogen. Int J Med Microbiol, 2007, 297(3): 197-204.

2. Krause PJ, Spielman A, Telford SR, et al. Persistent parasitemia after acute babesiosis. N Engl J Med, 1998, 339(3): 160-165.

3. Wormser GP, Prasad A, Neuhaus E, et al. Emergence of resistance to azithromycin-atovaquone in immunocompromised patients with *Babesia microti* infection. Clin Infect Dis, 2010, 50(3): 381-386.

4. Luo Y, Jia H, Terkawi MA, et al. Identification and characterization of a novel secreted antigen

1 of *Babesia microti* and evaluation of its potential use in enzyme-linked immunosorbent assay and immunochromatographic test. Parasitol Int, 2011, 60(2): 119-125.

5. Ooka H, Terkawi MA, Goo YK, et al. *Babesia microti*: Molecular and antigenic characterizations of a novel 94-kDa protein (BmP94). Exp Parasitol, 2011, 127(1): 287-293.

6. Tonnetti L, Thorp AM, Deisting B, et al. *Babesia microti* seroprevalence in Minnesota blood donors. Transfusion, 2013, 53(8): 1698-1705.

1.4 Zoonotic parasitic diseases

Parasitic zoonosis is a kind of disease caused by parasitic infections that are naturally transmitted between vertebrates and humans. According to incomplete statistics, there are almost 70 kinds of parasitic zoonoses, of which about 30 are common occurred in humans.[1]

Zoonoses are a group of important infectious diseases that severely endanger the health of people, livestock, and wildlife, as well as jeopardizing economic development. In recent years, the incidence of parasitic zoonoses shows an increasing trend in the world including China. In developed countries, where people live in highly urbanized environments, the incidence of human parasitic diseases has decreased to a very low level due to higher living standards. In developing countries, densely populated areas characterized by low living standards and poor sanitation lead to people having a higher chance of coming into contact with livestock, poultry, wild animals, and other pathogenic carriers. Thus, it is still relatively common that people suffer from parasitic zoonoses, making them to be an important global public health problem.

China is still a developing country, which suffers from zoonotic diseases. The Chinese government attaches great importance to the prevention and control of parasitic diseases in humans and animals. Remarkable achievements have been made in the research of etiology, diagnosis, treatment, prevention, and control. However, as zoonotic diseases can be transmitted in variety of ways, which are complex, affecting many humans and animals, it may be difficult to contain or eradicate these diseases in a short span of time. Currently, China faces the challenges of an increase of emerging zoonotic diseases and the return of reemerging ones.

Zoonosis can be classified based on biology and epidemiology, and also on route of infection or source of infection. When classified by biology, parasitic zoonoses can be divided into zoonotic protozoosis, trematodiases, cetodiases, nematodiasis, and epizoonoses.

More than 50 kinds of parasitic zoonoses have been reported in China, as shown in Table 1.7.[1, 2]

Table 1.7　Some of the parasitic zoonoses reported in China.

Classification	Species-specific infections
Zoonotic protozoosis	leishmaniasis, amebiasis, babesiosis, balantidiasis, sporidiosis, cryptosporidiosis, toxoplasmosis, giardiasis, and isosporiasis
Zoonotic trematodiases	schistosomiasis, clonorchiasis sinensis, paragonimiasis, fascioliasis, echinostomiasis, dicrocoeliasis, eurytremiasis, heterophyiasis, trichobilharziasis, Oriental bilharziasis, and cercarial dermatitis
Zoonotic cestodiases	taeniasis solium, cysticercosis cellulosae, taeniasis saginate, bothriocephaliasis, sparganosis, echinococciasis, coenuriasis, tenuicollis cysticercosis, dipylidiasis, hymenolepiasis, and raillietinasis
Zoonotic nematodes	toxocariasis, ancylostomiasis, trichinosis, strongyloidiasis, dirofilariasis, trichostrongyliasis, angiostrongyliasis, anisakiasis, gongylonemiasis, gnathostomiasis, thelaziasis, gordiasis, dioctophymosis, and ascariasis
Epizoonoses	myiasis, hirudiniasis, and sarcoptidosis
Other zoonoses	acanthocephaliasis, and linguatuliasis

In general, there is a lack of census and statistical data on most zoonotic parasites in China. The second national survey (2001–2004) of important human parasitic diseases examined several diseases.[3] It was found that the prevalence rate of leishmaniasis was 0.59% and its standardized prevalence rate was 0.49%. The seropositive rate of toxoplasmosis was 7.88% and its standardized seropositive rate was 7.97%. Both the infection and standardized rates of *Clonorchis sinensis* were 0.58%. The seropositive rate of paragonimiasis was 1.71% and its standardized seropositive rate was 1.70%; the highest standardized seropositive rate was in Shanghai (5.14%), followed by Chongqing (4.12%). The infection rate of *Taenia* spp. was very low throughout China, except for Tibet. The infection rate in Tibet was 21.08%, accounting for 86.98% of the total infections in the country. No infection of *Taenia* spp.

was found in 19 provinces, municipalities, and autonomous regions. Echinococcosis survey was carried out only in 12 provinces/autonomous regions where transmission presented, 10 of which are distributed in western China. The seropositive rate was 12.04% and its standardized seropositive rate was 11.98% detected by antibody-based serotests. The prevalence rate was 1.08% and its standardized prevalence rate was 1.12%, with echinococcosis cases detected by B-mode ultrasonography. The seropositive rate of cysticercosis was 0.55%, with 10 provinces/autonomous regions having a higher standardized seropositive rate. The rate of hookworm infection was 6.08%: the highest rate was in Hainan Province (34.58%), followed by Guangxi and Sichuan, with 19.67% and 18.01%, respectively. The infection rate of *Ascaris lumbricoides* was 12.57%; the highest was in Guizhou (41.59%), followed by Hunan (30.42%). By the end of 2013, 420 of the 454 schistosomiasis endemic counties (cities and districts) reached the standard of transmission control or transmission interruption. The other 34 counties were also at the stage of epidemic control, and were being promoted from epidemic control to transmission control.[4]

In recent years, with the development of the economy, the emerging veterinary industry has developed rapidly in China. The number of pet dogs, cats, birds, and fish has increased dramatically, and varieties have become more diverse. According to a 2007 report, the number of dogs in China was about 150 million.[5] The number of pet dogs, which require regular inoculation, medical treatment, and feeding with special dog food, is about 20 million. There were about 60 million domestic cats, from which eight to nine million were pet cats.

No systematic investigation has been conducted on the status of zoonoses in domestic animals or humans in China. The situation of the growing number of stray cats and dogs makes things even more uncertain. The number of pet dogs is growing by 10–20% every year.[6] Zoonoses related to pets and stray cats or dogs are of particular concern. But economic losses due to parasitic infection in animals are huge, up to more than billions of dollars annually.

References

1. Wang TP. Prevalence and Control of Parasitic Zoonoses. Chin J Parasitol Parasit, 2015, 33(6): 472-476. (In Chinese)

2. Qiu JH, Wang CR, Liu WT, et al. The species and epidemic situation of parasitic zoonoses in Heilongjiang Province as well as the measures of prevention and control. Heilongjiang J Animal Sci Vet Med, 2003, (6): 4-7. (In Chinese)

3. Technical steering panel for national survey of current status of major human parasitic diseases & office of national survey of major human parasitic diseases. Report on National Survey of Current Status of Major Human Parasitic Diseases in China. 269-295.

4. Lei ZL, Zhou XN. Eradication of schistosomiasis: a new target and a new task for the National Schistosomiasis Control Porgramme in the People's Republic of China. Chin J Schisto Control, 2015, 27(1): 1-4. (In Chinese)

5. Lin DG, Current Status. Opportunities and Challenges of Pet Industry in China. Chin J Comparat Med, 2007, 20 (11,12): 13-16. (In Chinese)

6. Zhou LS. The development prospect of pet industry in China. Guangdong J Animal Vet Sci, 2013, 38(1): 41-43. (In Chinese)

1.4.1   Schistosomiasis

Schistosomiasis is one of neglected tropical diseases (NTDs), and remains a major public health problem affecting many parts of the developing world. The main disease-causing species in humans are *Schistosoma japonicum*, *Schistosoma mansoni* and *Schistosoma haematobium*. It affects more than 200 million people worldwide and is endemic in approximately 70 countries, leading to the loss of 1.53 million disability-adjusted life years (DALYs).[1]

Schistosomiasis japonica, caused by infection with *S. japonicum*, was considered to be one of the most serious parasitic diseases endemic in China. The infection has been an epidemic for more than 2,100 years, as evidenced by a corpse (wife of a local authority) from the Western Han Dynasty found to have the presence of *S. japonicum* eggs by Chinese archaeologists in Mawangdui, Changsha, Hunan Province, in 1972. The first case report was published in the *Chinese Medical Journal* by Dr. Logon, an American medical doctor, who found a case administrated to the hospital in 1905, in Changde, Hunan Province. Since then, more and more field investigations and surveys have been carried out in this region surrounded by lakes and watercourses. It was estimated that about 12 million people are infected with *S. japonicum* in 12 provinces in China. Inhabitants of many places in south China have suffered from the disease, entering into vicious cycles of disease and poverty, due to its serious morbidity rate.[2]

Epidemiology

Efforts in the last six decades, supported by the Chinese government, communities, and experts in the control of schistosomiasis, have resulted into the efficient control of the disease in the entire country, with elimination achieved in many places. In 1955, Chairman Mao issued the statement: "we must eliminate schistosomiasis"; after which a vigorous national control program was established. As a result, schisto-somiasis japonica has been eliminated in five out of 12 provinces, including Shang-hai, Guangdong, Guangxi, Fujian, and Zhejiang. By the end of 2014, 98.90% of all endemic counties (448/453) had interrupted or controlled transmission of schisto-somiasis. However, the most difficult challenge is dealing with the remaining trans-mission areas of schistosomiasis japonica.

Due to several factors, for example, diversity and complexity of the ecological environment in endemic areas, increasing of snail dispersal after serious floods in 1998, and reduction of control efforts in endemic areas with comparatively weaker economic development, schistosomiasis has reemerged in 38 counties in seven prov-inces in 2001. The number of infected individuals reached 843,011 and 842,525 by the end of 2003 and 2004, respectively, and among them 1,114 and 864 were cases of acute infections, respectively.

Due to the schistosomiasis resurgence in 2004, China has redefined the disease control as one of the highest priorities in communicable disease control, together with human immunodeficiency virus infection and acquired immune deficiency (HIV/AIDS) and tuberculosis. To this end, a national program for schistosomiasis control has been initiated in 2004, by adopting a revised control strategy in order to strengthen the implementation of integrated measures aiming to reduce the transmis-sion of *S. japonicum*. The intensified national program was put forward for the five to ten year plan from 2008 to 2015. It aimed to control the transmission (prevalence rate both in humans and reservoir hosts less than 1%) by 2008, interrupt transmission by 2015 in both mountainous and plains regions, control the infection (prevalence rate less than 5% without any outbreak of acute infection) by 2008, and control the transmission by 2015 in lake regions.[3]

Control strategy

More than 50 years ago, China initiated the national schistosomiasis control program. With the ultimate aim of eliminating schistosomiasis, many approaches have been used, and the overall strategy has been adapted as new approaches and evidence emerged in response to the changing epidemiology of the disease. Three major strategies have been implemented at different stages:

- The early efforts from the early 1950s to later 1980s focused on the control of the intermediate host snails, and it was believed that schistosomiasis could be eliminated by chemical molluscicides and environmental management that targeted entirely snail habitats. Large-scale community participation was a central feature in environmental management. Although the snail habitats were substantially reduced and the number of human infections steadily declined, the disease remained difficult to eliminate on the way.

- Morbidity control was the backbone of the disease control in the 1990s, assisted by the administration of praziquantel, which had been introduced for large-scale use in the previous decade, coupled with health education. Schistosomiasis control was compliance with chemotherapy, which was dropped as the program evolved. This finding, coupled with factors such as severe flooding of the Yangtze River in the late 1990s, other ecological transformations, and forced movements of population, might explain the resurgence of schistosomiasis after the project was terminated. Indeed, the number of acute cases of human schistosomiasis and the snail-infested areas increased in the early 2000s.

- In view of the remaining challenges for sustainable control of schistosomiasis in China, a long-term action plan has been developed from 2004 to 2015, with the goals to (i) reduce prevalence of infection with S. *japonicum* to below 5% by 2008 (infection control), and (ii) decrease infection below 1% by 2015 (transmission control) in all endemic areas. To achieve these targets, the feasibility and cost-effectiveness of a four-pronged approach was investigated in different settings, with the aim of interrupting environmental contamination of schistosome eggs by humans and bovines. The four components are: (i) improved mechanization of agriculture to replace buffaloes with tractors; (ii) avoidance of marshland pastures and introduction of fenced cattle farming, as already done for pig farming; (iii) installation of sanitation facilities in houses; and (iv) provision of toilets for mobile populations (e.g. fishermen). The data from pilot studies as well as the actual program suggest that near-complete elimination of *S. japonicum* contamination is possible if such a multipronged strategy is integrated with other control activities. Importantly, such a strategy will not only be effective against schistosomiasis, but also against a range of other helminthic diseases (e.g. ascariasis, hookworm disease, and trichuriasis) that are still rampant in China. By the end of 2015, all endemic counties of the country have achieved the goal of transmission control, with a human infection rate of less than 1%. The central government of China has decided to continue this strategy to achieve transmission interruption by 2025.

Table 1.8 summarizes the lessons from 50 years of schistosomiasis control program in China, providing guidelines on long-term control and elimination of the disease to the global scientific community. However, to suit particular settings, the integrated strategy needs to be adapted. In addition, cost-effectiveness in different settings also needs to be investigated, so that schistosomiasis can eventually be eliminated as a public health problem not only in China, but also in other endemic countries.

Table 1.8   Lessons from 50 years of schistosomiasis control program in China.

Governmental policy
- Recognition of the public health significance of schistosomiasis
- Political will and commitment to control schistosomiasis

Control strategy
- Use of multiple interventions in an integrated way
- Adapt control interventions for specific ecoepidemiological settings and over time, as the challenge of control changes

Implementation, monitoring, and surveillance
- Rigorous surveillance and monitoring of human and bovine prevalence and snail-infested areas

Diagnosis

In general, *S. japonicum* can be diagnosed by three different approaches: (i) detecting schistosome eggs in fecal samples by direct parasitological methods and disclosing eggs in tissue biopsies by histological methods; (ii) testing immunological responses to certain schistosome antigens and the levels of parasite-derived antigens in blood and urine samples; and (iii) measuring pathological morbidity associated with schistosome infection by clinical, subclinical, and biochemical markers. There are other methods such as questionnaires, but their specificity is unproven.

Although the histological method is a sensitive and specific clinical diagnostic method, it is neither simple nor convenient for population-based surveys. There are many methods for measuring the morbidity and clinical morphological diagnosis associated with *S. japonicum*, but they lack in specificity.

Direct parasitological examination

Detection of parasite ova in stool is the traditional and still very widely employed diagnostic method for schistosomiasis infections. There are many variations of direct parasitological examinations, however, the Kato-Katz thick smear and the miracidium hatching test are the two widely field-applied methods of examining fecal samples for *S. japonicum* in China.

The Kato-Katz method is the most extensively used method for identifying *S. japonicum* eggs in field surveys because it is quantitative, relatively inexpensive, and simple. However, it has become quite insensitive following widespread chemotherapy, which results in generally lower worm burdens. The specificity and positive predictive value (PPV) of the Kato-Katz method are good irrespective of the adopted reference "gold standard" and the infection rate in humans. The sensitivities of this method vary from 40% to 100%, while the negative predictive values (NPVs) range from 52.5% to 100%. The last two parameters (sensitivity and NPV) of the Kato-Katz method are highly dependent on the infection prevalence among the population, and these two parameters generally decrease with the decrease of the infection rate in humans. For example, assuming two repeated Kato-Katz results as the reference "gold standard", the sensitivity of a single stool examination with a three-slide Kato-Katz method was 68.4–70.0% in Village A with an infection rate of 18.6%, and 59.6–69.2% in Village B with a prevalence of 6.6%, respectively. Thus, more than 30% of infected people will be misdiagnosed by the Kato-Katz method in endemic regions of China, and might therefore not get treatment, thereby continuing the transmission of schistosomiasis.

The Modulated Hydrothermal (MHT) is another traditional approach to assess *S. japonicum* infection, and has been used widely in China for more than five decades. The test is initiated by the concentration of ova from feces through a nylon tissue bag and suspension in distilled water. Miracidia that hatch from the ova are visualized microscopically, and their presence signals infection. The specificity and PPV of the MHT are high and identical irrespective of the adopted reference "gold standard" and the infection rate among the population. However, the sensitivities and NPVs of this method are wide ranging, from 24.0% to 95.0%, and from 40.91% to 99.62%, respectively.

The variational range of both the sensitivity and NPV of the MHT is larger than that of the Kato-Katz method. The result of the hatching test is unstable and significantly depends on the infection prevalence among the population and environmental factors such as temperature and water quality. For example, when the combined results of seven repeated Kato-Katz examinations and MHTs were used as the "gold standard", the sensitivity of the hatching was only 32.82% (less than 67.67% for a single Kato-Katz examination) in Zhuxi Village, while in Zhonjiang Village, the hatching resulted in more positive cases than Kato-Katz (prevalence of 31% versus 24%). This MHT has not been standardized for quantitative measurement and is not much more sensitive than Kato-Katz. More importantly, even under optimal conditions, only 50–70% of eggs will hatch, with light infections being missed.

Although multiple stool examinations should ideally be performed in order to reduce the number of false-negative results, repeated stool collection and examination requires a lot of time and human resources. Thus, it is impractical to initiate such a strategy at the national level for routine schistosomiasis control programs. As an ideal field method for the detection of schistosome eggs in stool is still not available, it is a challenge to demonstrate the presence of *S. japonicum* in the field.

Indirect immunological techniques

Indirect immunodiagnostic assays, that is, the detection of schistosome-specific antibodies, have a long history in China. There are many variations of indirect immunological methods, however, the circumoval precipitin test (COPT) and the indirect hemagglutination assay (IHA) are historically the most widely used immunodiagnostic tests in China, while various forms of enzyme-linked immunosorbent assay (ELISA) and dipstick dye immunoassay (DDIA) have become more important over the past 10–20 years.[4]

The COPT has been widely used in China for almost 50 years, and undergone a series of modifications including the application of a variety of labeling techniques in an attempt to standardize the testing system, including antigen preparation and testing protocol. The COPT has been shown to have a high sensitivity (94.1–98.6%) and low false-positive rate (2.5–3.6%) in healthy people from a non-endemic area. However, with repeated chemotherapy in endemic areas, the sensitivity of this method decreased to 72.2–85.8%. The NPV of this method is high (more than 87%), but the PPV is low (31.7–74.9%). In addition, it is time-consuming and comparatively complicated, and requires microscopy. These factors currently limit the method's wide application in China.

The IHA, with soluble extracts of schistosome eggs, was developed and applied in the late 1960s, and is secondary only to COPT in having been used for a long time in China. Currently, the IHA method is still extensively employed for community diagnosis and screening of people targeted for chemotherapy with praziquantel, due to its relatively high sensitivity, simplicity, and rapidity compared with the Kato-Katz and MHT methods. However, with repeated chemotherapy in endemic areas, most of the IHA's reported PPVs are less than 37%. The sensitivities of the IHA vary from 69.7% to 100.0%, and its specificities range from 35.7% to 93.6%. In addition, cross-reaction with *Paragonimus westermani* was shown to be 64–84% with soluble egg antigen (SEA) and 31.3% with purified egg antigen. These factors disturb the IHA method's continued wide application in China.

Enzyme-linked immunosorbent assay (ELISA) was first described by Engvall and Perlmann. In the late 1970s, the classic ELISA with crude antigens of the parasite emerged for the diagnosis of schistosomiasis. It was regarded as being most likely to meet stringent requirements for field use, as it was more reliable, sensitive, and specific. Soon after, many different variations of the basic theme have been developed for diagnosis (e.g. Dot-ELISA, SPA-ELISA). The sensitivities of this method vary from 65.5% to 100%, while the most reported specificities are less than 60%. The NPV of the ELISA method is high (>88.0%), but most of the reported PPVs are very low. Although this technique has relatively high sensitivity, an ELISA reader is required to process samples and the delay before it is possible to inspect the results is usually two to three hours.

The DDIA, a new immunodiagnostic assay, has been developed in recent years. This method is basically a chromatography technique using the SEA of *S. japonicum*, labeled with a dye. The sensitivity and NPV of the DDIA method are high (>75% for sensitivity, >94% for NPV), except for one report, in which the reference "gold standard". The specificity and PPV of this method show very large discrepancies; the specificity varies from 33.0% to 96.3% and the PPV ranges from 10.0% to 87.6%. In addition, the DDIA has a high cross-reaction with paragonimiasis (70.0%).

Although most of the reported sensitivities and NPVs of these antibody detection assays were relatively high, the discrepancy in both the reported specificities and reported PPVs was very large, and moreover, most of these reported specificities and PPVs were very low. The discrepancies attribute to the following factors: (i) the choice of the reference "gold standard"; (ii) infection prevalence and intensity in a community; (iii) different diagnostic agents of schistosomiasis; and (iv) size of the sample. Low specificity would result in a high "false seropositivity", that is, a high proportion of seropositive individuals were classified into the group with negative stool examinations in endemic regions, especially in areas with relatively severe endemicity, where reinfection and repeated chemotherapy are very common. For example, the false-positive rate of IHA was 44.21% in a village with a prevalence of 18.63%, and 32.77% in another village with a prevalence of 6.62%, while that of ELISA was higher (61.63%), when the two accumulated Katz-Kato results were designated as the "golden standard". Apart from the low specificity and PPV, these assays generally have a high cross-reaction with other parasites (e.g. *P. westermani*). Among all obstacles of antibody-based immunodiagnostic tests, the major one is that these currently available assays cannot distinguish active infections from previous infections or reinfections, which results in a high false-positive rate. This limitation causes difficulties in determining prevalence, identifying infected individuals for selective chemotherapy, and assessing the effectiveness of the intervention.

Direct immunological tests

Immunoassays have shown that schistosome-derived antigens were present in the circulation and/or excreta of infected hosts, and these observations prompted considerable research on their potential for immunodiagnosis of schistosomiasis. In the early 1980s, research was initiated by Qian and Deelder to explore the detection of the circulating anodic antigen (CAA) [5] for the immunodiagnosis of *S. japonicum* infection in China. The results demonstrated that the detectable limit was from 10 to 0.5–0.25 ng/mL using the CAA series. Thus far, many testing systems based on monoclonal or polyclonal antibodies for the detection of different target antigens have been developed in more than 10 laboratories in China.

In 1993, a collaborative study focusing on evaluation testing systems for antigen detection was conducted in China. The results showed that most of the tests involved in the detection of different circulating antigens were not performed properly, with high false-positive sero reactivity ranging from 24% to 46% and low sensitivity ranging from 15% to 73%. Afterwards, a special national program initialed under the supervision of the Schistosomiasis Expert Advisory Committee, Ministry of Health of China. It aimed at improving the diagnostic capacity of existing assays and seeking novel probes, with an emphasis on those that could be promising in the monitoring of the efficacy of chemotherapy. Then, in 1995, fourteen testing systems (thirteen for antigen detection and one for antibody detection) from twelve laboratories were brought to Wuhan City for a collaborative evaluation. Among the thirteen assays for antigen detection, nine showed high specificity (above 90%), however, only three assays had a rate of above 68% for sensitivity, of which the highest one was 81%, in chronic and light infections. Furthermore, there was no clear-cut evidence that antigen-based assays could provide useful correlation to levels of infection intensity.

It is very difficult to select diagnostic methods for *S. japonicum* infections in areas where reinfection and repeated chemotherapy are frequent. On the one hand, if every person found positive with antibody-based immunodiagnostic assays is treated with praziquantel year after year, a considerable number of previous infections will be treated repeatedly, which results in abuse of praziquantel and a reduction of chemotherapy compliance. On the other hand, if these immunodiagnostic assays are only used for preliminary screening, and all those with positive results are subjected to stool examination to confirm infection, then only individuals with positive rates of egg count are treated, and a higher proportion of infections will be missed. It must be concluded that the insensitivity or non-specificity of currently applied diagnostic methods conspire to produce inaccurate estimates of disease impact, and this threatens the successful drive towards full control of schistosomiasis. Hence, a search for a good diagnostic test that can be applied in field situations is essential and should be given high priority.

Treatment

The antimony potassium tartrate treatment was first used in clinical practice in 1918. By the 1970s, the development of praziquantel and its widespread use in the 1980s resulted in the incidence and mortality rates of schistosomiasis decreasing significantly.[6] However, any drug may produce a significant decrease in the incidence and death rate of schistosomiasis. Any kind of drug can also produce drug resistance. In recent years, in order to solve the problem of praziquantel resistance and anti-drug resistance, a lot of work has gone into searching for an alternative to praziquantel, which is broad-spectrum, and has a high efficiency and low toxicity.[7]

Praziquantel is a well-known broad-spectrum, anti-parasitic drug.[8-9] After being developed in 1979, it became the first choice for treating schistosomiasis and other parasitic diseases, also playing a major role in the control of fluke and tapeworm disease. Praziquantel has low toxicity in humans and animals, and is also considered to be suitable for the treatment of children and pregnant women. Praziquantel can rapidly destroy the skin of the insect and invade the body. The mechanism is still uncertain and may be the activation of the insect's body.

Oxamniquine, one of the four tetrahydroquinoline derivatives developed in the late 1970s, is the most promising schistosomicide.[10] Praziquantel and oxamniquine are different. Praziquantel is not valid for *S. japonicum* in Brazil and other South American countries.[11,12] Oxamniquine is the main drug used to treat schistosomiasis mansoni; the ratio of male and female *S. mansoni* killed by oxamniquine is 2:1, oxamniquine is invalid for schistosomula.[13]

Unlike praziquantel, an important feature of artemether is the ability to induce the reinfection of *S. mansoni*. Bergquist and colleagues reported that artemether triggers mice to efficiently resist reinfection of *S. mansoni* and produces the same level of reinfection with *S. mansoni* as those produced by irradiated cercaria. So far, no resistance of artemisinin to schistosomiasis has been reported, or even a widely used antimalarial drug. Due to the low cure rate of praziquantel in high infection areas, artemisinin may be the most useful anti-schistosomiasis drug.

Recently, it has been found that mefloquine might show anti-schistosomiasis activity in mice.[14,15] To treat *S. mansoni* or *S. japonicum* infection in schistosomula and adult mice, they are administered a 200–400 mg/kg single oral dose of mefloquine, causing female parasites to greatly reduce or even disappear. In mice infected with *S. mansoni* that were administered a slightly lower dose of 150 mg/kg of mefloquine, the amount of spawning was significantly reduced. Keiser's study further demonstrated that mefloquine can quickly kill the adult worms of *S. japonicum* in the body. Studying the mechanism of fluquin against schistosomiasis, Zhang and colleagues confirmed that the killing rate of fluquin is very fast, and its mechanism is to induce insecticidal action by inducing histopathological changes in some tissues and organs. The effect of mefloquine on female schistosomes is stronger than on male ones. Further studies have shown that, at the same dose, the effect of mefloquine on *S. japonicum* adult worms is better than praziquantel.

In 1963, Niridazole was the first drug to be developed for oral anti-schistosomiasis. Besides anti-schistosomiasis activity, it also inhibits the action of cell immunity and anti-amoeba protozoa. Niridazole not only presents anti-*schistosoma haematobium* activity, but also exhibits activity in relation to *S. mansoni* and *S. japonicum*; the effect of the former is, however, better than the latter two. The mechanism may be an inhibition of *Toxoplasma gondii* glucose-6-phosphate dehydrogenase activity, increased body glycogen utilization, and glycogen depletion. It can also degenerate the genitals of its flukes.

Niridazole is used to treat schistosomiasis, as it has a good killing effect on adults. The possible mechanism of its action is that the body of three carboxyl cycle metabolism is disturbed, resulting in lack of energy supply body, which finally leads to death. The effect on the schistosomula child is weaker than on the adult, and a larger dose can prevent it from developing into adult.

References

1. Steinmann P, Keiser J, Bos R, et al. Schistosomiasis and water resources development: systematic review, meta-analysis, and estimates of people at risk. Lancet Infect Dis, 2006, 6: 411–425

2. Zhou YB, Song L, Jiang QW. Factors impacting on progress towards elimination of transmission of schistosomiasis japonica in China. Parasit Vectors, 2012, 5: 275

3. Yang GJ, Sun LP, Hong QB, et al. Optimizing molluscicide treatment strategies in different control stages of schistosomiasis in the People's Republic of China. Parasit Vectors, 2012, 5: 26.

4. Tu JL, Jiang CF, Zhang YJ, et al. Detecting effect comparison between MPAIA, DDIA and IHA for screening advanced schistosomiasis. Zhongguo Xue Xi Chong Bing Fang Zhi Za Zhi, 2012; 24(6): 729-30. (In Chinese).

5. Corstjens PLAM, Hoekstra PT, de Dood CJ, et al. Utilizing the ultrasensitive *Schistosoma* up-converting phosphor lateral flow circulating anodic antigen (UCP-LF CAA) assay for sample pooling-strategies. Infect Dis Poverty, 2017; 6(1): 155.

6. Li YS, McManus DP, Li DD. et al. The schistosoma japonicum self-cure phenomenon in water buffaloes: potential impact on the control and elimination of schistosomiasis in China. Int J Parasitol, 2014, 44(3-4), 167-171.

7. Webster BL, Diaw QT, Seye MM, et al. Praziquantel treatment of school children from single and mixed infection foci of intestinal and urogenital schistosomiasis along the Senegal River Basin: monitoring treatment success and re-infection patterns. Acta. Trop, 2013, 128(2), 292-302.

8. Li H, Dong GD, Liu JM, et al. Elimination of schistosomiasis japonica from formerly endemic areas in mountainous regions of southern China using a praziquantel regimen. Vet Parasitol, 2014, DOI: 10.1016/j. vetpar.

9. Doenhoff MJ, Pica-Mattoccia L. Praziquantel for the treatment of schistosomiasis: its use for control in areas with endemic disease and prospects for drug resistance. Expert Rev Anti-Infet, 2006, 4, 199-210.

10. Sabah AA, Fletcher C, Webbe G, et al. *Schistosoma mansoni*: Chemotherapy of infections of different ages. Exp Parasitol,1986, 61, 294-303.

11. Xiao SH, Yue WJ, YangYQ, et al. Susceptibility of Schistosoma japonicum to different developmental stages to praziquantel. Chin Med J, 1987, 100, 759-768.

12. Botros S, Sayed H, Amer N, et al. Current status of sensitivity to praziquantel in a focus of potential drug resistance in Egypt. Int J Parasitol, 2005, 35(7), 787-791.

13. Blanton RE, Blank WA, Costa M, et al. *Schistosoma mansoni* population structure and persistence after praziquantel treatment in two villages of Bahia, Brazil. Int J Parasitol, 2011, 41(10), 1093-1099.

14. Keiser, J.; Chollet, J.; Xiao, S.H. Mefloquine-an aminoalcohol with promising anti-schistosomal properties in mice. PloS. Neglect Trop Dis, 2009, 3(1), e350.

15. XiaoSH, Mei JY, Jiao PY. Further study on mefloquine concerning several aspects in experimental treatment of mice and hamsters infected with *Schistosoma japonicum*. Parasitol Res, 2009,106(1), 131-138.

1.4.2   Echinococcosis

Echinococcosis (also called hydatid disease or echinococcal disease) is a parasitic disease that affects both humans and other mammals such as sheep, dogs, rodents, and horses. There are two different forms of echinococcosis found in humans, namely, cystic echinococcosis caused by *Echinococcus granulosus*, and alveolar echinococcosis caused by *E. multilocularis*. These are caused by the larval stages of different species of the tapeworm *Echinococcus* spp.[1]

Epidemiology

Hydatid disease is more prevalent in the northern hemisphere. Human infection is most common in sheep-raising countries such as Australia and New Zealand, the Middle East, Russia, South America, North Africa, North China, Mongolia, and Japan.[2]

Echinococcus granulosus is endemic in at least 21 provinces, autonomous regions, and municipalities in China, covering approximately 87% of the country's territory. The highest prevalence occurs in seven provinces/autonomous regions, including Xinjiang Uygur Autonomous Region, Tibet Autonomous Region, Ningxia Hui Autonomous Region, Gansu Province, Qinghai Province, Inner Mongolia Autonomous Region, and Sichuan Province.

Echinococcus multilocularis is distributed mainly in the western and central parts of mainland China, including regions such as Xinjiang Uygur Autonomous Region, Qinghai Province, Ningxia Hui Autonomous Region, Gansu Province, Inner Mongolia Autonomous Region, Sichuan Province, and Tibet Autonomous Region.

Sporadic human cases have also been reported in the northeastern parts of Heilongjiang Province.[2]

In China, new cases of hydatidosis have increased since 2004, with six people dying in 2007 (Figure 1.3, Table 1.9).[5]

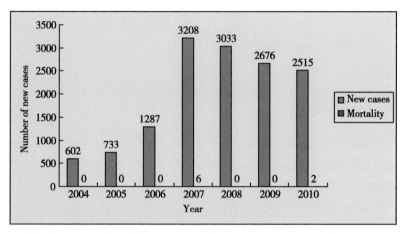

Figure 1.3   The repartition of the number of hydatidosis cases in China, 2004-2010.

Table 1.9   New case reports of hydatidosis in China during 2002-2010.

Disease	Hydatidosis	
Year	Case reports	Number of deaths
2002	–	–
2003	–	–
2004	602	0
2005	733	0
2006	1,287	0
2007	3,208	6
2008	3,033	0
2009	2,676	0
2010	2,515	2

Control strategy

Hydatidosis is defined as a category C of the notifiable infectious disease, and a regular surveillance network has been established. The Ministry of Health of China issued the "Action Plan for the Control and Prevention of Hydatid Disease (2010–2015)" in 2010, in order to promote the national echinococcosis control programme into a high agenda of government.

Diagnosis

The diagnosis of cystic echinococcosis includes several steps, which were well described in the World Health Organization (WHO) technical report[2]: suspicion on clinical grounds or upon screening confirmed by imaging (CT, X-ray, etc.) and identification of characteristic or suspicious cyst structures, which is confirmed by the detection of specific antibodies through immunodiagnostic tests, e.g. enzyme-linked immunosorbent assay (ELISA), Immunofluorescent assay (IFA), immunoblot, detection of "Arc 5" antibodies, etc. Diagnostic puncture may be considered in cases where there is doubt of infection, if it is not contraindicated. Material obtained by biopsy puncture or surgery can be examined, such as hydatid fluid for Echinococcus protoscoleces or hooks, protoscoleces for DNA by polymerase chain reaction (PCR), antigen from sterile cysts, and cyst wall material for characteristic structures by histological study.[2]

Diagnosis of alveolar echinococcosis is based on similar criteria, that is determining case history including epidemiological hints, clinical findings, morphological lesions detected by imaging techniques, and immunodiagnostic tests.

In addition to pathogen detection methods, immunodiagnostic kits also play a crucial role. A query lodged through the Chinese Food and Drug Administration (China FDA) website (http://www.sfda.gov.cn/WS01/CL0001/) yielded that China currently has four approved hydatid disease diagnostic kits: two are ELISA kits for the detection of anti-echinococcus immunoglobulin (IgG) antibodies and two are colloidal gold kits for the detection of hydatid disease antibodies.

Recently, researches on diagnostic methods for echinococcosis have mostly been based on serology testing. Chen and colleagues produced the recombinant antigen B (rAgB) and compared its serodiagnostic activity with natural antigens using the dot immunogold filtration assay (DIGFA). Their results showed that rAgB can improve specificity but decrease sensitivity, and they believed that the combination of native and recombinant antigens can improve the overall performance of cystic echinococcosis serodiagnosis.[3] Wang and colleagues showed that an immunochromatographic test using crude hydatid cyst fluid and a recombinant 18-kDa protein (rEm18) is a good tool for the simultaneous detection and discrimination of both cystic and alveolar echinococcosis, and is useful for the serodiagnosis of both types in clinical settings and screening programs.[4] Liu et al. found that the first diagnostic suspicion is usually based on a hepatic ultrasound exam performed due to abdominal symptoms or in the context of a general checkup; hydatid alveolar echinococcosis (HAE) diagnosis may thus also be an incidental finding on imaging. The next step should be a CT or magnetic resonance imaging (MRI).[5] Gao and colleagues established and evaluated a colloid gold immunochromatographic strip test for the diagnosis of alveolar echinococcosis. This strip was firstly prepared using RNA from *E. multilocularis* protoscoleces and an Em18 gene was obtained by reverse transcription PCR. Then, the PCR product was sequenced, cloned, and expressed as a recombinant protein. The developed immunochromatographic strip test using the recombinant Em18 antigen as a coated antigen is a sensitive, specific, simple, and rapid assay for diagnosing alveolar echinococcosis.[6] In another study, five subunits of the echinococcus antigen B (AgB) family were analyzed and the sensitivities of the subunits for cystic echinococcosis sera were obtained. This study proved that the paralogous subunits EgAgB1, EgAgB2, and EgAgB4 were the main reactive subunits in sera detection and may have utility as echinococcosis diagnostics, with EgAgB1 showing the greatest potential. Moreover, the cocktail subunits may improve the positive detection rate.[7] A new three-minute dot (dot immunogold filtration assay [DIGFA]) for serodiagnosis of human cystic and alveolar echinococcosis was developed in 2010. This simple eye-read rapid test can be used for both clinical diagnostic support, as well as in conjunction with ultrasound for mass screening in endemic cystic and alveolar echinococcosis areas.[8]

Literature review on echinococcosis diagnosis studies conducted in China

In order to review the progress on researches of echinococcosis diagnosis in China, the China National Knowledge Internet (CNKI) and Wanfang databases, two of the most important academic websites, were searched in Chinese and the major progress are summarized as follows:

Searching in CNKI (http://www.cnki.net/) with 'diagnosis of *Echinococcus hydatid*'/+ theme/keyword queries (Table 1.10), a total of 1,996 literatures were yielded, and 114 most relevant records were collected and analyzed. Among them, the five journals that published most papers on this topic are *Chinese Journal of Parasitology & Parasitic Diseases* (53%), *Journal of Ningxia Medical College* (3.5%), *Xinjiang Medical University Journal* (3.5%), *Animal Husbandry and Breeding Science* (3.5%), and *Modern Biomedical Progress* (2.6%). The research institutions mainly cited are the National Institute of Parasitic Diseases at China CDC for (6.1%), the First Affiliated Hospital of Xinjiang Medical University (6.1%), the Xinjiang Medical University (5.3%), People's Hospital of Xinjiang Uygur Autonomous Region (4.4%), and Qinghai University Affiliated Hospital (3.5%). Research funding came from Chinese grants of the National Science Foundation (7%), the National High-Tech Research and Development Program (1.8%), the National Science and Technology Support Program (1.8%), the Cheung Kong Scholars Program (0.9%), and the Qinghai Province Science Foundation (0.9%).

Table 1.10   Query results from CNKI and Wanfang databases.

Keywords	CNKI	Wanfang
Endemic	170	233
Survey	153	294
Site	32	5
Screening	19	10

A total of 916 results were obtained when searching for specific keywords of echinococcosis diagnosis in China. Among them, there were 170 and 233 publications about endemic studies on echinococcosis in CNKI and Wanfang databases, respectively. Of all the searched publications, 153 and 294 were on field surveys, 32 and five were concerned with survey site; and 19 and 10 were associated with population screening, respectively.

In the top 100 relevant articles, it was found that the most popular diagnostic methods used were B-mode ultrasonography and ELISA. Table 1.11 summarizes all of the results.

Table 1.11　Diagnostic reagents/methods mentioned in publications.

Diagnosis reagents/methods	Number
ELISA kit	16
DIGFA	2
B-mode ultrasonography	18
Antigen rapid filtration method for rapid diagnosis	1
Rate stem IFA	1
Indirect hemagglutination assay (IHA)	1
PCR method	4
Western blot	1
Intradermal test	1
ELP antigen	1
Total	**46**

References

1. https://en.wikipedia.org/wiki/Echinococcosis#cite_note-0#cite_note-0

2. Eckert J, Gemmell MA, Meslin FX, et al. WHO/OIE manual on echinococcosis in humans and animals: a public health problem of global concern. Office International des Epizooties, Paris, 2001.

3. Chen X, Chen X, Lu X, et al. The production and comparative evaluation of native and recombinant antigens for the fast serodiagnosis of cystic echinococcosis with dot immunogold filtration assay. Parasite Immunol, 2015, 37(1): 10-15.

4. Wang JY, Gao CH, Steverding D, et al. Differential diagnosis of cystic and alveolar echinococcosis using an immunochromatographic test based on the detection of specific antibodies. Parasitol Res, 2013, 112(10): 3627-3633.

5. Liu W, Delabrousse É, Blagosklonov O, et al. Innovation in hepatic alveolar echinococcosis imaging: best use of old tools, and necessary evaluation of new ones. Parasite, 2014; 21: 74.

6. Gao CH, Shi F, Wang JY, et al. Establishment and evaluation of colloid gold labeled immunochromatographic strip test for rapid diagnosis of alveolar echinococcosis. Zhongguo Ji Sheng Chong Xue Yu Ji Sheng Chong Bing Za Zhi, 2012, 30(2): 90-94.

7. Jiang L, Zhang YG, Liu MX, et al. Analysis on the reactivity of five subunits of antigen B family in serodiagnosis of echinococcosis. Exp Parasitol, 2012, 131(1): 85-91.

8. Feng X, Wen H, Zhang Z, et al. Dot immunogold filtration assay (DIGFA) with multiple native antigens for rapid serodiagnosis of human cystic and alveolar echinococcosis. Acta Trop, 2010, 113(2): 114-120.

1.5 Responding to outbreaks of parasitic diseases

Parasitic diseases can potentially cause long-term harm to people's health. Although outbreaks of parasitic diseases are less frequent than they used to be, such as *Schistosoma japonicum* infection in China during the 1950s and 1960s, they may still lead to serious harm. As there has often been a lack of effective emergency response approaches and techniques in the outbreaks of some rare emerging parasitic diseases, there is an urgent need to gather information on the actual situation regarding this issue in China.

1.5.1 Determinants of parasitic disease outbreaks and history of exposure

The primary task is to verify the disease outbreak as soon as possible. Epidemiological investigation should be rapidly conducted. In order to estimate whether the number of cases exceeds expected judgments, the history of clinical cases and epidemiological information should also be carefully verified in the epidemic area.

Three factors are of particular importance: (i) human factors: if the number of cases reported to increase or decrease, for instance, changes were caused by diagnostic methods; the promotion of health education publicity has increased people's awareness of health as well as decreased the infection rate; due to the increasing number of migrant workers, the number of imported parasites also increased; (ii) statistic factor: whether there was a statistical significance in the number of increasing cases compaired the previous data; (iii) circumstance factor: whether there was an association between cases in time or space, for example, before the establishment of the People's Republic of China, the people's living standards as well as medical and health levels were poor, and the number of parasitic infections was high. With the establishment and reform, and opening up of China, the people's living standards have gradually improved, the sanitary conditions have been improved, the medical level has been greatly improved, and the parasitic infection rate has dropped significantly.[1]

1.5.2 Confirmation of indicator cases

Epidemiological survey

Epidemiological surveys can provide an important basis for the diagnosis of parasitic diseases. The specific content of these survey include the following:[2, 3]

- An understanding of local geography; the seasonal distribution of rainfall; the nature and quantity of arable land; soil and vegetation characteristics; and animal populations and distribution.
- Investigation of the number of patients, their sex and age, eating habits, food sources, quality of water and living conditions, etc.
- Survey on the presence and distribution of the intermediate host and vector.

Clinical detection

Clinical detection involves observing the unique clinical symptoms of some parasitic diseases, such as pivotal movement in cerebral echinococcosis, and itching of cercariae dermatitis and hair removal from the skull in the infection on mite. For atypical symptoms, clinical detection can also determine the degree of harm and the main manifestations of a disease. Furthermore, it can provide a basis for diagnosis by other methods.[4]

Detection of pathogens in laboratory

Many methods to detect pathogens can be undertaken in a laboratory, taking different materials from distinct parasites. The main methods are:[4]

- Stool examination, including morphological detection of parasite in fecal sample, egg detection, miracidia hatching, and the larvae inspection method. As eggs and oocysts of parasites are excreted with feces, stool examination is therefore one of the most important means of diagnosing parasitic diseases.
- Skin scrapping materials (dander) detection: this method is suitable for the laboratory diagnosis of mite infections.
- Blood test, which is used to diagnose blood parasitic infections, such as *Plas-*

modium, *Toxoplasma*, and *Babesia* infections. Thin and thick blood smears are always applied.

- Urine detection: it is mainly used in egg tests for *Schistosoma haematobium*, whose eggs can pass through the vein wall into the bladder and are excreted in the urine.

- Genital secretion, which is mainly used for trichomoniasis diagnosis.

Other laboratory examination methods include the anus wipe examination, sputum and nasal lymph fluid examination, and biopsy material inspection. If necessary, animal inoculation experiments should be carried out, which is often the case for some protozoan pathogens, such as trypanosomiasis and toxoplasmosis.[4]

Therapeutic diagnosis

Suspected patients are treated with the proven effective medicine for that specific parasitic disease.

- Helminthicide diagnosis: Helminthicide is carried out using a specific effective drug, and feces are collected after deworming within three days. Parasites in feces are observed by the naked eye to determine their number and species. This method is suitable for the diagnosis of teniasis, nematodes, and other intestinal parasites.[5-8]

- Treatment diagnosis: An effective drug is used in the treatment of suspected patients, according to the treatment effect. The effect is assessed according to the symptoms, and body condition (e.g. improved, healing). This has mainly been used in the diagnosis of protozoa and worms in organs and tissues.

Immunological detection

Common immunological diagnostic methods include: circumoval precipitin test (COPT), indirect haemagglutination assay (IHA), enzyme-linked immunosorbent assay (ELISA), immunofluorescent assay (IFA), latex agglutination (LA) test, Western blotting, and immunochromatographic technology.[9]

Molecular diagnosis

Molecular diagnostic techniques mainly include DNA arrays and polymerase chain reaction.[9-12]

1.5.3   Confirmation of transmission scope and intensity

Baseline survey

The baseline survey collects detailed demographic data, such as living environment, customs, economic development, as well as weather information. The aim is to understand the population's health status, education/production activities, population movements, and other information.[13, 14] The prevalence of natural foci of the disease as found in previous studies should be highlighted.

Case survey

The objective of the case survey is to include cases and suspected cases by conducting a cross-sectional study and historical analysis, combining field investigation with laboratory testing. It requires the collection of information on the basic circumstances surrounding the case, after the onset of disease, and clinical and epidemiological history before the onset. The survey of initial cases and indicator cases should be highlighted. The epidemiological associations between initial cases should be analyzed, indicating cases and consecutive cases, analyzing chains of transmission, and investigating and analyzing severe and fatal cases. Meanwhile, the survey group and test group must establish closely contact with each other to understand the working procedures.[15] In order to guarantee the provision of high-quality laboratory samples, field staff have to be clearly aware of the type of laboratory samples required (blood/fecal/sputum/urine), the acquisition methods (etiology, serology or molecular biology), and storage and transportation conditions (room temperature, −20 degrees Celsius frozen under or frozen in liquid nitrogen).[4] When suspecting the outbreak was new-onset natural foci parasitic disease, it should try to strengthen the mortality, reproductive index basis, spread rate and other key indicators. These are early indicators to assess the strength and danger of epidemics important warning parameters.[16]

Survey of intermediate hosts and vectors

If suspecting that an outbreak is a new-onset natural foci parasitic disease where no special parasitic disease appearing before (in a certain area, diseases that can be transmitted without human beings, but can be transmitted to humans through certain animals as hosts), landscape ecology and the natural features of landscape development, operation, control type, population density, and seasonal growth and decline of local host animals and vectors should be investigated systematically.[17] There should also be a comprehension of the possible route, frequency, and intensity of parasitic disease outbreak when exposed to wild animal hosts and vectors, and a knowing of wildlife hunting, selling, and processing. Human, animal, or poultry serum, and/or tissue samples in endemic areas should be collected systemically. Suspicious host animals and/or vectors should be targeted for carrying out the relevant pathogen detection.[16]

Etiological analysis and verification

After survey data are verified, major indicators and parameters should be dynamically analyzed.

The focus should be on the species and quantities of hosts and vectors; etiology and serology results; three distribution factors (population, time, and space); frequency and mutual exposure; the incidence time series; and other indicators. In order to determine any significant differences between the main indicators and parameters, the possible reasons for these differences must be analyzed as well as a mathematical analysis conducted, and so on.

Confirmed analysis by clinical, laboratory, and epidemiological data on the assumption of parasitic disease, including the causative agent exposure history, the possible cause of outbreaks, pathogenic features, and popular feature of consistency. Moreover, surveys can be conducted or supplementary investigations can be expanded on. Further, case-control or cohort studies can be carried out, in particular historical cohort studies on the etiology of hypotheses.

Disease prevention and control

Timeliness is critical in an outbreak investigation and response. Control measures should be synchronized with the cause of assumptions made, without waiting for hypothetical verification, in order to avoid delays in control. Once the assumptions of how the parasitic disease outbreaks are made, immediate measures against the hypothesis should be taken. Moreover, control measures should be synchronously modified.

General control measures against epidemics include three links, focusing on the source of infection and high-risk populations. The foci of ecological control measures in a unique position and role in the natural foci of disease outbreaks disposal site, are of concern. For example, in schistosomiasis epidemic areas, composting and fermenting of cattle manure is required to kill eggs and prevent the spread of schistosomiasis.

According to the cause of judgment, combined with the disease incubation period, the number of vulnerable people exposed and exposure cases (especially severe or fatal cases), treatment, disease progression and outcome, should be estimated.[17]

1.5.4　Emergency response strategies and measures

The establishment of emergency response agencies

When an outbreak occurs, depending on the severity of the epidemic and hazard rating, the appropriate government should quickly set up emergency headquarters; if the outbreak is limited to a certain area, this is usually done by the region's Department of Health. Emergency response members typically include health administrative department heads, clinical doctors, experts of zoonoses, epidemiologists, specialists of infectious diseases, media specialists, biology specialists, veterinary science experts, and, if appropriate, ecology and food inspection experts.[17] An emergency response agency would include an epidemiological survey group, test group, medical group, prevention group, as well as logistics, security, and other advocacy groups, as needed. Each group should strengthen inter-group cooperation, carry out epidemiological investigations, take appropriate control measures to coordinate the treatment of patients, establish and verify the reason of outbreak, and notify and report outbreak disposal in a timely manner.[16]

Disease reporting and information dissemination

According to disease severity and development, and control, the emergency agency reports to the national government, through initial reports, periodic briefings, and summary reports. The summary report includes the event name, type and nature, location, time of occurrence, number of cases and deaths, major clinical signs and symptoms, possible causes, measures taken, and the effect of epidemic development trends. After a preliminary investigation is conducted, an epidemic alert should be issued as soon as possible to provide timely and accurate early warning information to the public. If appropriate, a helpline should be established. Clear epidemic content should be posted to local hospitals and a person in charge of response should be designated. Information by any other organization or individual should not be released without authorization. If the outbreak involves many regions, the regions should closely coordinate with each other.[16]

1.5.5 Response assessment

During an outbreak of a parasitic disease, according to the epidemiological investigation and pathologic examination, a dynamic analysis should be carried out on trends and the implementation of control measures.

After implementing the emergency treatment plan in epidemic areas, there will be a significant reduction in new cases. The number of cases will decrease to the same level or even lower as compared to previous years within a month, which can be regarded as the control of a preliminary outbreak. It can then be transferred to routine control and monitoring.

1.5.6 Case reports

Case report 1: Emergency response to a trichinosis outbreak in Lanping County, Yunnan Province

On March 4, 2009, ten human poison cases were reported, including three severe cases (one case was fatal) in Lanping County, Yunnan Province. As trichinosis was suspected, in order to verify the cause and control the further spread of the epidemic, experts from the Chinese Center for Disease Control and Prevention (China CDC) and Yunnan Provincial CDC went to the epidemic areas to carry out an epidemiological survey, pathogenic detection, and serum test. The nature and extent of the epidemic was accurately determined, thus the outbreak was kept under control.

Stage I: Response to the incident

(1) Outbreak

On February 18, 2009, nine people in Biyu River Village, Lanping, Yunnan, presented with symptoms of fever, headache, nausea, vomiting, abdominal pain, diarrhea, muscle pain, and body swelling, following by limb weakness, muscle tension, and joint stiffness. This incident was reported as "mass poisoning incidents". By February 27, one person died.

(2) Epidemiological investigation

On March 3, an epidemic survey, and pathogenic and serum detection were carried out by five experts from the China CDC and Yunnan Provincial CDC. The investigation included clinical and etiological diagnosis of cases (the common meal history of workers and the surrounding population, including family members and residents of the village). The sources of infection of livestock and other subjects were also detected to verify the diagnosis. A case survey was also conducted, potential cases were tracked and investigated, and the source of infection was traced.

(3) Response

a. Pathogenic and serum detection: A gastrocnemius examination of six patients found that four cases were infected with *Trichinella* larvae. In the serological detection of nine patients, eight had an immunoglobulin (Ig) G/IgM positive result. It was decided that the outbreak was incident trichinosis.

b. Epidemic investigation: After treatment with albendazole, symptoms of the nine patients markedly improved. A case study (see below) was conducted among the nine patients, who had varying degrees of headache, nausea, aching limbs, limb weakness, and other symptoms typical of the onset of trichinosis.

- Case study on a preliminary analysis:
  - Incidence of time distribution: The first case showed symptoms on January 15; late onset cases were on February 14. The outbreak mainly happened between January 15 and 20, and February 1 and 14.
  - All ten patients were road workers on the Zhonggong local road.

○ All ten patients were male. The youngest was 17 years old and the oldest was 55 years old. Seven patients aged 20–50 years.

● Assumptions:

○ The infection occurred among people with a common history of eating together, especially in minority people.

○ The population lives surrounding the areas where the patients infected with trichinosis live.

○ There was a potential infection source in local areas, for example, the outbreak occured during the transmission season of schistosomiasis, increased risk of human infection in areas where host snails or cattle are concentrated

c. Expanded investigation conducted among the surrounding population and tracing the source of infection: There were 17 workers who ate together (which included the ten infected patients, one of whom died). Besides the infected patients, one worker could not be contacted as he was working in the mountains. Among the other six people, serological detection and health education were conducted. The serological detections were all negative.

The investigation of the population living in surrounding areas included serological detection being carried out among 22 family members of the patients and villagers. A total of five people had a positive result in the IgG test, and one showed a positive IgM reaction.

Tracing the infection source found that the pork eaten by the patients came from a pork butcher, Shuhong Yang. Serological detection was done on another pig and it was positive. Furthermore, in order to investigate the situation of the pork supply site, samples of pork from Heqing and Eryuan Counties were collected. The detection results were all negative.

d. Health education: Informing the risk of eating raw or uncooked meat and introduce the hazards of trichinosis through promotional materials.

Stage II: Investigation of the cause

Four aspects contributed to the outbreak. The first was the poor self-protection awareness of local people. Local people did not understand trichinosis transmission and harm. Village pigs were mostly bred in the backyard. Family health status was poor, regardless of raw and cooked cooking cutting board, which led to the larval of *Trichinella* attached to cutting board. Second, parasitic disease prevention and treatment level of local professionals were low. The local government and medical institutions should increase the publicity of the disease and inform the villagers how to prevent infection. Third, the local medical equipment was outdated.

Stage III: Response evaluation

(1) Verification of pathogenic and serological detection

With the combination of clinical symptoms of nine patients and epidemic history, pathogenic and serological detection supported that the outbreak was due to the common eating pork infected with *Trichinella spiralis*.

(2) Epidemiological investigation

There was a potential infection source in the local area. Although health education was administered, changing eating habits is a long and arduous process.

Case report 2: Response to an outbreak of human *Fasciola gigantica* in southwest China

Outbreak[18]

Twenty-nine hospitalized patients from 18 families were distributed in four adjacent townships (Zhoucheng Town and neighboring communities) in the south part of Binchuan County, Yanman Prevince. Two families reported four cases each and five families reported two cases each, which indicated family clustering of fascioliasis. Only six patients from three families complained that they had a dinner together in late September 2011. The other families did not report sharing dishes in the late half of 2011.

Epidemiological investigation

Due to the insidious onset and long illness course, the exact date when the patients were attacked by fascioliasis was difficult to determine. Instead, the potential date was inferred according to clinical records and findings from the 1:1 matched case-control study. The peak occurred in late November 2011, and there was a second peak of hepatalgia in late January 2012. It was notable that pain in the liver in most of patients was generally dull and many patients were not aware of such discomfort until their condition deteriorated. Furthermore, one male adult did not report hepatalgia during the entire illness course.

Responses

(1) Clinical examination

Among 29 cases, 65.5% patients were female. Moreover, only two patients were less than 20 years old and the median age was 35 years old. Twenty-two cases were farmers.

Due to intermittent fever lasting a few months, 27 patients went to hospital for diagnosis and treatment. However, the remaining two were febrile after admission. The intensity of fever was moderate, but could exceed 41°C, and was of irregular character. Hepatalgia occurred in almost all patients with the exception of one male adult. Epigastric pain and percussion sensitivity in the liver affected 89.7% and 62.1% of the patients. Only 10 patients showed hepatomegaly and three more did so during hospitalization. Some patients experienced weight loss.

A series of biochemical indicators regarding liver and kidney function were detected. The level of alkaline phosphatase (ALP) and γ-glutamyl transpeptidase (GGT) were sharply elevated. The levels of ALP and GGT also increased in 65.5% and 86.2% of the patients. Only two patients and one patient showed normal levels of ALP and GGT, respectively, during their hospitalization, due to obstruction in the biliary system.

However, the indicators reflecting cholangitis and jaundice/bilirubin (BIL) and total bile acid (TBA) showed different profiles. Almost all patients appeared normal in terms of total BIL and indirect BIL. An increase in direct BIL was observed in 44.8% of the patients. TBA was elevated in 69.0% of the patients. However, only one patient showed a constant increase for all indicators. Therefore, it was referred that the major hepatic lesion might be obstruction in bile canaliculus, which induced a high ALP and GGT, but not a high BIL and TBA.

The most significant indicators for the damage of hepatic cells are alanine aminotransferase (ALT) and aspartate aminotransferase (AST). Five patients showed a constant increase for both levels in all indicators. Furthermore, the levels of ALT and AST increased simultaneously in two patients, which implied that there were no matches in the change of such two indicators. Five patients also appeared as having normal levels of ALT and seven appeared as having normal levels of AST. Therefore, the disease in these patients was not as severe as implied by the manifestations of hepatic cellular damage.

In 27 patients, there was a constant increase in their C reactive protein (CRP) level, which signaled that the disease was in the acute stage. In contrast, the ratio of albumin and globin significantly declined. Significant changes were observed in lactate dehydrogenase, alpha-hydroxybutyrate dehydrogenase, creatine kinase, and cholinesterase.

White blood cell count increased in the patients. The majority of patients showed a high eosinophil count or the proportion in the whole illness course. In terms of red blood cells (RBCs), 48.3% of the patients showed a declined count and 37.9% showed a fluctuation. The remaining four showed normal RBC counts. Decreasing levels of hemoglobin and hematocrit were commonly observed in the patients. Moreover, most of the patients showed a fluctuation in platelet during their illness course. An increased erythrocyte sedimentation rate was observed in 14 out of 15 patients.

Hepatic lesions by B-mode ultrasonography and computed tomography (CT) were used to examine all patients. Typical imaging showed many low-density masses with irregular shapes, which indicated the winding migration route in the liver and inflammation. Moreover, another common finding in imaging examination could be splenomegaly. Twenty-three patients had an enlarged spleen. In addition, 16 and 17 patients were found to have ascites and hydrothorax, respectively.

Except for the pathological change described above, a hepatic biopsy was performed on two severe cases, by laparoscopy. Convex nodes of 0.5–1.5 cm in diameter on the liver's surface were observed in one patient. The sections from isolated tissue showed a mixed necrotic structure with tunnel-like lesions and small colliquative lacuna. Around the lesions were eosinophils, lymphocytes, and plasma cell. Charcot Leyden crystals could be seen by staining. No definite worm structures were found.

(2) Treatment diagnosis

It was confirmed that *F. gigantica* was the pathogen in these patients' infection. First, symptoms and findings from supplementary examinations were consistent with fascioliasis. The most significant indicators included increased eosinophil count, manifestations and images regarding hepatic lesion, and intermittent fever. Second, a series of differential diagnoses had been made to exclude bacterial and viral infections, as well as other potential helminth infections. Third, broad-spectrum, anti-parasitic drugs (e.g. albendazole, mebendazole, levamisole, praziquantel, and artemether) failed to control the illness. Triclabendazole was successful for treatment. Fourth, the seroprevalence of *F. gigantica* (100%, 26/26) was higher than that of *F. hepatica* (80.8%, 21/26). Moreover, a significantly higher relative optical density (OD) of the former (1.70) than the latter (1.18) was observed ($P < 0.05$). Last, *Fasciola* eggs were obtained from the fecal samples of four patients. The eggs measured 153–175 × 75–95 μm, which was consistent with the dimensions reported for *F. gigantica* (150–196 × 90–100 μm), but not for *F. hepatica* (130–150 × 63–90 μm). Furthermore, the eggs were confirmed by nuclear and mitochondrial gene sequences.

After confirming diagnosis, the rest of the patients were administrated triclabendazole with an oral dosage of 10 mg/kg/day for two successive days. Although the biochemical and cellular indicators did not go normal soon after, the conditions of patients improved significantly 4–5 days post-treatment; fever especially was controlled satisfactorily. No notable side effects due to triclabendazole were reported by patients.

The potential sources of infections were explored. Freshwater vegetables (i.e. watercress, wild rice stem, lizard tail, and scallion) were commonly consumed. There was no significant difference between the consumption of these vegetables in patients and controls. Few patients or controls ate raw watercress and water bamboo. However, lizard tail and scallion were commonly consumed raw. It was noted that there are two distinct types of lizard tail on local markets, i.e. shoot with leaves and bare root. The former was produced locally and normally eaten raw. By contrast, bare roots were generally imported from other places and also consumed raw, but were occasionally fried. However, no obvious difference was observed. Farmers grew lizard tail in water fields and fertilized it with feces of domestic animals. Meanwhile, many intermediate hosts, freshwater snails (*Galba* spp.), were found in the fields.

(3) Serological and molecular detection

Twenty-seven serum samples were obtained from the patients. All samples were detected intensively against the crude antigen of *F. gigantica*. Moreover, 57 family members of patients were also diagnosed by serological test, with 26.3% of these having a positive result. In contrast, only 8.8% of 3,177 participants beyond the patients' families were found to be serologically positive. As the former was significantly higher than the latter (*P*<0.05), this supported a family clustering of fascioliasis. Although a total of 279 participants were serologically positive, only three had *Fasciola* eggs in their stool samples.

Molecular identification was also done by amplifying internal transcribed spacer (ITS) + and cytochrome c oxidase subunit 1 (cox1) sequences of *Fasciola* spp. from seven patients (including three cases identified in extensive epidemiological investigation), 40 cattle, 10 goats, and one snail. Then, the phylogenetic relationship was reconstructed by NJ analysis of cox1 sequences. The examined specimens were clustered into two major clades of these samples. The big one included *F. gigantica* and most of the examined egg samples from patients, cattle and goats, and snails. The second one contained *F. hepatica*, and five samples from cattle and four from goats.

(4) Expanded investigation

There were 468 cattle and 104 goat stool samples from 13 communities collected, with a 28.1% prevalence. No significant difference was observed between cattle (28.6%) and goats (26.0%). In terms of aquatic snails, 2,437 of these belonging to three genera, i.e. *Radix*, *Physa*, and *Galba*, were detected for *Fasciola* spp. infections in snails Only one collecting site was inhabited by infected snails. Cercariae within snails were confirmed by a genetic marker. There were no trematode species in 2,412 snails from the other 35 sites.

References

1. Binder S, Levitt AM, Sacks JJ, et al. Emerging infectious diseases: public health issues for the 21st century. Science, 1999, 284(5418): 1311-1313.

2. Guo CS. Epidemiological investigation and emergency disposal of public health emergencies. Modern Med and Health Res, 2004, 38 (1): 65-67. (In Chinese)

3. Li YL. Human Parasitology (Seventh Edition). Beijing: People's Health Publishing House, 2009. (In Chinese)

4. Garcia LS, Arrowood M, Kokoskin E, et al. Laboratory Diagnosis of Parasites from the Gastrointestinal Tract. Clin Microbiol Rev, 2017, 31(1).

5. Leber AL (ed). Clinical microbiology procedures handbook, 4th ed. ASM Press, Washington DC, 2016.

6. Garcia LS (ed). Clinical microbiology procedures handbook, 3rd ed. ASM Press, Washington DC, 2010.

7. Hinz R, Schwarz NG, Hahn A, et al. Serological approaches for the diagnosis of schistosomiasis - A review. Mol Cell Probes, 2017, 31: 2-21.

8. Zheng Z, Cheng Z. Advances in Molecular Diagnosis of Malaria. Adv Clin Chem, 2017, 80: 155-192.

9. Zhang JF, Xu J, Bergquist R, et al. Development and application of diagnostics in the National Schistosomiasis Control Programme in the People's Republic of China. Adv Parasitol, 2016, 92: 409-434.

10. Weerakoon KG, McManus DP. Cell-free DNA as a diagnostic tool for human parasitic infections. Trends Parasitol, 2016, 32(5): 378-391.

11. Binnicker MJ. Multiplex Molecular panels for diagnosis of gastrointestinal infection: performance, result interpretation, and cost-effectiveness. J Clin Microbiol, 2015, 53(12): 3723-3728.

12. Chen ZS. Epidemiological investigation and emergency treatment measure of public health emergencies. Chin Health Standard Manag, 2016, 7(11): 6-7. (In Chinese)

13. Wang JL. Discussion of epidemiological investigation and emergency disposal of public health emergencies. Today Health, 2015, 14(2): 317. (In Chinese).

14. Gratz NG. Emerging and resurging vector-borne diseases. Annu Rev Entomol, 1999, 44: 51-75.

15. Sun MZ. Crisis management disposal and strategie of emergency public health. Fudan University Press, 2013. (In Chinese)

16. Russell K, Addiman S, Grynszpan D, et al. The impact of new national guidance for the public health management of enteric fever in England. Public Health, 2017, 154: 79-86.

17. Marano N, Pappaioanou M. Historical, new, and reemerging links between human and animal health. Emerg Infect Dis, 2004, 10(12): 2065-2066.

18. Chen JX, Chen MX, Ai L, et al. An Outbreak of Human *Fascioliasis gigantica* in Southwest China. PLoS One, 2013, 8(8): e71520.

Chapter 2

Malaria in China

**Bin Jiang, Jun Feng, Xiao-nong Zhou, Guo-jing Yang,
Zhi Zheng, and Zhi-bin Cheng**

2.1 Introduction

Malaria is a mosquito-borne infectious disease caused by the eukaryotic protist of the genus *Plasmodium* via the bite of a positive female *Anopheles* mosquito. Four *Plasmodium* species, including *Plasmodium falciparum*, *P. vivax*, *P. malariae*, and *P. ovale*, have been found in China (Figure 2.1). Among them, the most common ones are *P. falciparum* and *P. vivax*, with proportion rates of 58% and 42%, respectively. *Plasmodium falciparum* is the most fatal one.

2.1.1   History of malaria transmission in China

Historically, China suffered seriously from malaria epidemics. Malaria has been documented in traditional Chinese medicine books, and the presence of malaria goes back approximately 4000 years in China's history.[1] Malaria expanded broadly, especially in rural regions, and outbreaks occurred often over the last few decades. According surveillance report, malaria has been widespread in China, with 24 malaria-endemic provinces and over 24 million cases being reported in the early 1970s. The Chinese government launched the national malaria elimination pro-gramme in May 2010, aimed at reducing the number of locally transmitted malaria cases across most of China to zero by 2015 (except in some border areas of Yunnan province where the goal is elimination by 2017), and achieving World Health Organization (WHO) certification of malaria elimination for China by 2020.

From the foundation of the People's Republic of China in 1949 to reaching the goal of malaria free in 2020, the transmission patterns of the disease can be grouped

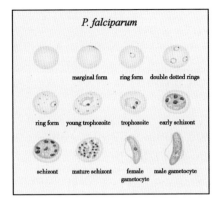
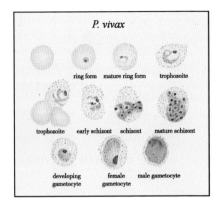
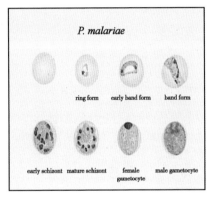
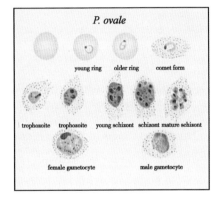

Figure 2.1 Species of *Plasmodium* found in China.

into five phases: (i) transmission not known (1949–1959); (ii) outbreak and pandemic transmission (1960–1979); (iii) decline with sporadic distribution (1980–1999); (iv) low transmission with re-emergence in central China (2000–2009) ; and, (v) the elimination phase (2010–present).[2]

Prior to 1949, there were approximately 30 million cases of malaria reported in China annually, and the mortality rate was about 1%. After control efforts were intensified in China in 2007, the incidence of malaria was substantially reduced in the provinces with malaria transmission, with 95% of these counties (2,345/2,469) having an estimated incidence below 1 per 10,000 persons in 2009. With the implementation of an integrated strategy for malaria control after 1980s, including interventions, as well as socio-economic and environmental development, such as urbanization, alterations in the natural surroundings which affected the transmission pattern including changes of malaria vector distribution, the occurrence of indigenous malaria cases has been steeply reduced, and epidemic regions have drastically shrunk.[3] Compre-hensive intervention policies and strategies have been much strengthen after malaria elimination programme was launched in 2010, the total number of malaria cases was remarkably reduced, in 2017 zero indigenous malaria infections was reported in all 24 provinces of China where malaria was epidemic.[2]

2.1.2   Current status of malaria in epidemiology

Currently, malaria is a mandatory notifiable infectious disease on the list of class B notifiable diseases as according to the Law on the Prevention and Control of Infec-tious Diseases in China.

Based on the report from surveillance system, the malaria incidence was fluctu-ated before 1980 at high level (Figure 2.2), with effective measures, such as diag-nosis, treatment, surveillance, health education, malaria cases have decreased from 24 million in 1970s to 200,000 in 2008. From 2006, malaria started to reemerge in the central and southern provinces where the disease used to be highly endemic with the incident rate of 0.49/10,000. Since 2007, imported malaria cases have become

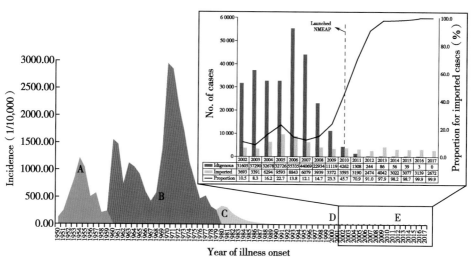

Figure 2.2   Incidence of malaria in China, 1950–2017. The different control and elimination phases are shown in different colors. (A) transmission not known (1949–1959); (B) outbreak and pandemic transmission (1960–1979); (C) decline with sporadic distribution (1980–1999); (D) low transmission with re-emergence in central China (2000–2009) and (E) the elimination phase (2010–2020). The indigenous and imported cases from 2002–2017 are shown in the right column.

a major issue due to a large number of Chinese workers coming back home from abroad. While in 2010, a total of 7,855 cases were reported with the incidence rate of 0.6/100,000, including 4,262 local infections and 19 deaths, and the 97 local falciparum cases were only reported in Yunnan province.

The patterns of indigenous malaria cases

The data from 2004 to 2017 indicated 204,859 local malaria (76.4%) and 63,329 imported malaria (23.6%) cases. During this period, the local transmission was sharply decreased by 99.9% from 2004 ($N = 32,678$) to 2016 ($N = 3$). And in 2017, no indigenous case was reported throughout the whole country. Indigenous cases were mainly documented in two regions since 2014, and only in 2 counties from 2 provinces in 2016. From 2005 to 2016, most indigenous cases (92.5%) were reported in Anhui ($N = 2,326$ [38.8%]), Yunnan ($N = 1,375$ [22.9%]), Henan ($N = 930$ [15.5%]), Hubei ($N = 459$ [7.7%]), and Guizhou ($N = 458$ [7.6%]). In recent years, the local vivax malaria in China was mainly reported in two regions, the counties along the border of China-Myanmar and Motuo County of Tibetan Autonomous Region, while the local *P. falciparum* only occurred in the border counties of Yunnan Province.[4]

The distribution of mosquito vector

The residual transmission by 2015 might reflect the spatial variability and complexity of *Anopheles* vectors in China. Among the counties with only *An. sinensis* and/ or *An. lesteri* as dominant vectors, the number of *P. vivax* and *P. falciparum* cases decreased substantially, with only one county reporting the occurrence of locally transmitted *P. vivax* in 2015. However, among the counties with other dominant vectors (e.g. *An. minimus, sensu lato (s.l.)*, *An. dirus s.l.*, *An. stephensis*, and *An. maculatus*), there were still more than 10 counties (with a combined population of about 3,766,000) reporting locally transmitted *P. vivax* annually in 2013–2015, and two counties (with a combined population of 569,000) reporting locally transmitted *P. falciparum* in 2015.[5]

The patterns of imported malaria cases from 2011 to 2015[5]

A total of 15,840 (89%) imported malaria cases were reported from 2011 to 2015 (see Figure 2.2). All 31 provinces reported cases, with a median of 3091 cases per year (interquartile range, IQR: 3,049–3,221 cases). The imported cases originated from 69 countries (44 in Africa, 18 in south-east Asia and seven in other regions). Most imported cases were among males (14,972; 95%) and Chinese nationality migrant workers (14,849; 94%). The median stay was longer in Africa (320 days; IQR: 171–515) than in south-east Asia (120 days; IQR: 59–229).

Most cases imported from Africa (8,756/10,949; 80%) were infected with *P. falciparum*, whereas a high proportion (3,362/4,340; 78%) of cases from south-east Asia were due to *P. vivax*. The majority of cases from south-east Asia were imported to Yunnan Province (3,082; 71%), whereas cases from Africa were mostly imported to Guangxi (1,834; 17%), Jiangsu (1,603; 15%) and Sichuan (884; 8%) provinces. For *P. vivax*, 1,536 counties (54% of all 2,858 counties) only reported imported cases, six counties (0.2%) only reported locally transmitted cases and 18 counties (0.6%) had both. For *P. falciparum*, 857 counties (30%) only reported imported cases, 90 counties (3%) only reported locally transmitted cases and 103 counties (4%) had both.

How to maintain the free status of malaria transmission

Based on the aforementioned characteristics of malaria transmission in China, the most challenge for the national malaria elimination programme is that how to maintain the free status of malaria transmission and prevent reintroduction in areas where malaria transmission has been interrupted. Therefore, the elimination programme is also need in couple with the social-economic development, which could respond to the malaria eradication initiative from the United Nations SDGs. In responding to the call of global malaria elimination by the World Health Organization (WHO), the Chinese government launched the National Malaria Elimination Action Plan (2010–2020) in 2010, which intends to eliminate indigenous malaria by 2020. However, with the economic development in China, the globalization, e.g. global transport, global investment, global human resource, etc., becomes a challenge for malaria elimination, as imported cases of *P. falciparum* malaria increased by 49.13% in non-endemic provinces and the number of deaths was 30 in 2011, which was double as the number in 2010. Therefore, technically, surveillance and response system is need further strengthened in the elimination and post-elimination era in order to maintain the free statues of malaria transmission.

References

1. Yin JH, Zhou SS, Xia ZG, et al. Historical patterns of malaria transmission in China. Adv Parasitol. 2014; 86: 1-19.

2. Feng J, Zhang L, Huang F, et al. Ready for malaria elimination: zero indigenous case reported in the People's Republic of China. Malar J, 2018; 17: 315.

3. Hu T, Liu YB, Zhang SS, et al. Shrinking the malaria map in China: measuring the progress of the National Malaria Elimination Programme. Infect Dis Poverty, 2016; 5(1): 52.

4. Feng J, Xiao H, Xia Z, et al. Analysis of malaria epidemiological characteristics in the People's Republic of China, 2004–2013. Am J Trop Med Hyg, 2015; 93(2): 293-9.

5. Lai S, Li Z, Wardrop NA. Malaria in China, 2011-2015: an observational study. Bull World Health Organ, 2017; 95(8): 564-573.

2.2 National Malaria Control and Elimination Programme

2.2.1 Control strategy

Evaluation of control strategy in the history

Malaria, one of the most important human parasitic diseases globally, has a significant impact on not only the health of the affected populations, but also the social and economic development of the areas where it is prevalent. In China, more than 30 million malaria cases were recorded annually during the 1940s and the mortality rate was about 1%. After the foundation of the People's Republic of China, the Chinese government paid a lot of attention to the severe malaria situation and invested a significant amount of resources into the malaria control program.[1] This led to a big improvement in the control of the disease (Figure 2.3), and as a result, today, most of the country is free from malaria. In 2010, only 7,855 cases were reported in a few provinces, and transmission of *P. falciparum* was confined to only two provinces.

From 2002 to 2012, China successfully awarded by Global Fund to Fight HIV/AIDS, Tuberculosis and Malaria (GFATM) for five grants dedicated to malaria control, such as: Round 1 (R1), Round 5 (R5), Round 6 (R6), Round 10 (R10) and

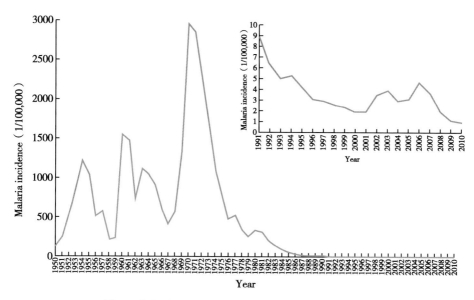

Figure 2.3   Malaria incidence in China, 1950–2010.

the National Strategy Application (NSA). The last grant reflected the shift from a rounds-based mode to an ever closer alignment with the National Malaria Elimination Programme (NMEP). Overall, approximately 116 million USD had been disbursed by the GFATM for these grants. The coverage of GFATM-supported projects gradually expanded from 47 counties in 2003 to 762 counties in 20 provinces in 2010.[2] GFATM malaria programme R1 covered 25 border counties of the Yunnan province, 10 counties of the Hainan province and 12 counties of the other 8 project provinces or autonomous regions (including Henan, Hubei, Anhui, Jiangsu, Guangdong, Guangxi, Sichuan and Guizhou). The target area for R5 covered 6 provinces, namely Yunnan, Hainan, Anhui, Henan, Hubei and Jiangsu provinces. Overall, 19.14 million people at risk living in rural areas of 1813 townships in 121 counties benefited directly and a further 63.8 million benefited indirectly from the activities. GFATM malaria programme R6 covered 12 counties in Yunnan province of China and 4 special administrative regions in Myanmar on the China-Myanmar border. GFATM malaria programme R10 covered 5 special regions in Myanmar on the China-Myanmar border and seven border counties in Yunnan. The target population included 586,000 local residents and 100,000 Chinese migrant workers in Myanmar as well as 1.5 million frequent border crossers.[2]

In China, great achievements on malaria control have been gained, for example, the malaria incidence decreased from 4 per 10,000 to below 1 per 10,000 over the past 10 years. As the biggest international cooperation programme focusing on malaria in China, the GFATM malaria programmes was instrumental in this success, which has produced tremendous impacts in the following six fields, including (i) promoted the national malaria control programme transited from malaria control to elimination in China, (ii) filled up the resource gap for malaria control and elimination, (iii) improved the multi-sectorial cooperation and communication, (iv) contributed to the policy making and ability of the national malaria control and elimination, (v) enforced public awareness of malaria control and prevention, (vi) established the cross-border cooperation mechanism for malaria control. In terms of declining the malaria burden in China significantly contributed by the GFATM malaria programmes, much lower transmission of malaria has been observed in 2011, the annual reported malaria incidence in 88% of the 75 Type 1 counties was less than 1 per 10,000, and 21.33% of Type 1 counties and 86.17% of the 687 Type 2 counties reported zero locally transmitted malaria cases. Over the 10-year period, most notably in the frame of R1, R5 and NSA, *P. falciparum* malaria was eliminated in Hainan province. The incidence in target counties of Hainan was 0.4 per 10,000 in 2007, and in 2011 there were no locally transmitted *P. falciparum* malaria cases. In Yunnan, the *P. falciparum* malaria incidence dropped significantly year by year and was close to 0.12 per 10,000 in 2011 (Figure 2.4).[3] What technical anti-malaria measures implemented and contributed to the malaria burden declined significantly in this period of time, it has been noticed that malaria control and elimination policy in the fields of diagnosis, treatment and vector control were revised over the course of implementation of the GFATM malaria programmes. As new malaria control techniques such as rapid diagnosis tests (RDTs), long-lasting insecticide treated nets (LLINs) and artemisinin-based combination therapies (ACT) were introduced to China, these new techniques were integrated into the national malaria control policy and well implemented to the entire country.

With the social-economic development in China, China's political commitment to health system reform has been put into its highest level of government agenda since 2006, that all Chinese people should have access to affordable essen-

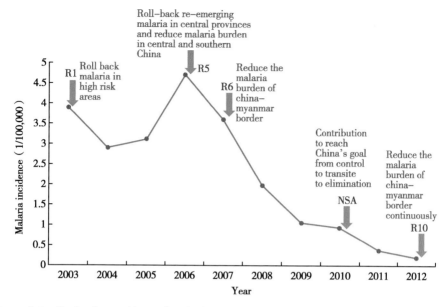

Figure 2.4 Reduction pattern of malaria incidence correlated to the rounds of GFATM malaria programmes in 2003–2012.

tial health services. A steady disease control and prevention system was established and strengthened, and human resources for health were increased through systematic training and continuing education courses. These laid the most important basis for the achievements of malaria control in China. Given the remarkable success achieved in the national malaria control programme (see Figure 2.3) and confidence that China can achieve even more, the national expert committee on malaria of China summarized experiences in malaria control and developed to the revised National Malaria Control Strategy in 2006, with the ambitious goal of elimination of malaria in China (*Handbook for Malaria Control and Prevention*). This revised strategy centered on a new stratification based on malaria transmission status at the county level. As shown in Figure 2.4, counties were categorized into four types according to local malaria incidence rates in 2006–2008.[3] In order to achieve elimination, interventions and activities were carefully designed to be effective, comprehensive, locally appropriate, equitable, sustainable, and feasible. With the support of other partners and governmental sectors, efforts were made to achieve the stated goals. These efforts were very much aligned with those of the United Nations Millennium Development Goals, the global fight against malaria as expressed in the Global Malaria Action Plan 2008, and the Regional Action Plan for Malaria Control and Elimination in the Western Pacific (2010–2015).

The WHO proposed that once malaria incidence is less than 1 case per 1000 population at risk annularly, a malaria elimination programme could be initiated. Since 1990, China's average malaria incidence rate at the country level has decreased to 1 per 10,000 annually. However, some locations are still heavily epidemic in specific ecosocial zones, with some outbreaks occurring from time to time. For instance, a malaria outbreak occurred in northern Anhui province in 2006. The Chinese NMEP was not launched until 2010, with the aim to eliminate malaria nationwide by 2020. Nevertheless, taking consideration of the fact that transmission patterns and elimination capacities vary from county to county, malaria elimination strategies need to be identified based on local settings, such as at the county level in different phases of the national programme.

In the history of the national malarial control programme in China, the stage-based malaria control strategy was adopted based on epidemiological patterns in local settings. The elimination strategy applied in the NMEP was also formulated based on the transmission patterns in different phases. More stages of the elimination programme exist in the classification of the Chinese NMEP compared to the WHO classification. Therefore, more detailed elimination strategies are identified for each stage in the Chinese NMEP. For instance, from pre-elimination to post-transmission, there are only three phases in the WHO classification—the pre-elimination phase, the elimination phase and the post-transmission phase—until certification of malaria elimination in 3 years. The elimination phase is normally much longer, usually more than 5–10 years. Therefore, Chinese classification uses five stages, which are based on the indices of malaria transmission and control capability (Table 2.1).[4]

2.2.2 Malaria elimination strategy

Implementation of malaria surveillance and response

The surveillance and response system is well integrated within the public health system in China, and all effective and prompt malaria response measures depend on timely and accurate information provided by the surveillance system. The relevant information is filtered, verified, stored on dedicated web-based platforms, and then disseminated and analysed by end users. Depending on epidemic data, vector data and other

Table 2.1 Comparison of various strategies in the WHO and Chinese classifications.

WHO classification	Preelimination	Elimination	Postelimination
Annual incidence	Slide or rapid diagnostic test positivity rate <5% in fever cases	<1 case per 1,000 population at risk/year	Zero locally acquired cases for 3 years
WHO strategy	Reinforcing the coverage of goodquality laboratory and clinical services, reporting and surveillance aimed at halting transmission nationwide. Perfecting the quality and targeting of case management and vector control operations, and introducing/maintaining activities aimed at consistently reducing the onward transmission from existing cases in residual and new active foci. Establishment of a strong surveillance system, with the cooperation of all healthcare providers.	Identification and treatment of all malaria reservoir and reduced transmission by vectors with full surveillance for clearing up malaria foci and reducing the number of locally acquired cases to zero. Identifying and treating all malaria cases with efficacious antimalarial medicines against liver stage and blood stage parasites, including gametocytes. Reducing human–vector contact and the vectorial capacity of the local Anopheles mosquito populations in transmission foci by efficacious vector control, personal protection and environmental management methods.	Maintain an effective surveillance and response system and strengthen prevention and management of imported malaria to prevent introduced cases and indigenous cases secondary to introduced cases. Reduction of vulnerability population. Screening of immigrants for malaria and the use of radical treatment in places where importation of malaria is intensive.

Continue

Chinese classification	Stage E1	Stage E2	Stage E3	Stage E4	Stage E5
Annual incidence	>1/1,000	1/1,000–1/10,000	<1/10,000	0	0 locally acquired case for successive 3 years
Chinese strategy	Strengthening infection control integrated with vector control measures Improving control capabilities to reduce the risk of transmission.	Strengthening training to improve local abilities. Appropriately control infection source to consolidate malaria control efforts.	Strengthening the surveillance response system Finding and treating imported cases earlier.	Strengthening surveillance, both active and passive surveillance, for early detection of infection sources.	Strengthen the surveillance response system to prevent the reintroduction of malaria cases.

relevant data acquired through surveillance system, the malaria response system is capable of completing the investigation and verification of individual cases, screening surrounding populations and implementing relevant vector control strategies.

In China, the national malaria surveillance was established in the beginning of the national malaria control programme in the 1950s, and further intensified with an official document issued by Ministry of Health in 2005. At early stage, the country was in the malaria control stage, with the objective to reduce malaria incidence and mortality. According to a survey in 2003 supported by the GFATM, the malaria incidence in the whole country amounted to 740,000 of cases, and hundreds of millions of people were at risk of malaria infection in 907 counties/cities/prefectures in 18 provinces/autonomous regions/municipalities (P/A/M). As a result, a total of 62 surveillance sites were set up in 2005, covering in 18 P/A/M of the country where conducting surveillance in key monitoring areas. Since 2010, when the country declared it was entering the malaria elimination stage, the epidemiological features have changed significantly. Under the NMEP, not only the target but also the strategies and measures in the elimination stage are significantly different from those in the control stage. The surveillance and response to individual case and focus is the vital strategy and key interventions in the elimination stage. Consequently, the country initiated the national surveillance system under NMEP in 2012, which consists of both routine surveillance and sentinel surveillance. Sentinel surveillance sites were selected based on malaria incidence and entomological considerations, categorized into two types of sites: sites with more local cases and sites with more imported cases.

Surveillance as an intervention in the NMEP

China's surveillance system for malaria elimination comprises routine surveillance and sentinel surveillance at three administrative levels: (i) the national level, conducting by the National Institute of Parasitic Diseases, Chinese Center for Disease Control and Prevention (CDC); (ii) the provincial level performing by provincial disease control and prevention agencies; and (iii) the county level, implementing through the county CDC where the surveillance site is located. The routine surveillance that covers the whole country includes daily case reporting, checkup and case investigation of malaria cases, including specific activities such as case verification, active case detection, blood examination and missing report investigations at regular intervals. Sentinel surveillance is focused on those activities that cannot covered by the routine surveillance system in all counties, such as entomological surveillance (species, density), drug resistance monitoring and insecticide resistance surveillance.

The national malaria elimination surveillance sites (hereinafter referred to as the national surveillance sites) cover 25 P/A/M. A total of 49 national malaria surveillance sites have been set up by county/city/district as a unit and divided into two categories according to their degree of malaria prevalence and characteristics. One category is for areas with more local malaria cases, including the following eight P/A/M: Anhui, Guizhou, Hainan, Henan, Yunnan, Hubei, Tibet and Jiangsu. Twenty-nine counties/cities/districts with relatively higher local malaria incidence in the most recent 3 years were selected as surveillance sites. The other category is for areas with more imported malaria cases, including Beijing, Shanghai, Zhejiang, Fujian, Shandong, Liaoning, Guangxi, Guangdong, Henan, Hunan, Jiangsu, Anhui, Sichuan, Chongqing, Hebei, Shanxi, Jiangxi, Shaanxi, Gansu and Xinjiang. Twenty counties/cities/districts with relatively more imported malaria cases in the most recent 3 years were selected as surveillance sites.

The nationwide routine surveillance mainly includes five activities: case reporting, diagnosis checkup, case investigation, active case detection and blood examination of unexplained fever cases. Sentinel surveillance consists of two scenarios: one scenario is focused on local transmission; the activities involved blood examination of unexplained fever cases, serological antibody test, entomological surveillance, insecticide-resistance surveillance and drug-resistance surveillance of *P. falciparum*. The other scenario is targeted to malaria importation, in which the surveillance activities comprise sentinel hospital surveillance, returned overseas screening and drug-resistance surveillance of imported *P. falciparum*.[5] Data collection is through an internet-based system, namely the National Information Management System for Malaria, and an annual surveillance report is released to the public in the form of white books or online papers.

Lessons shared from control strategy

Strategy formulation supported by implemental research

All of process for control strategy formulation was fully supported by implemental and evidence-based research. The archived facts, such as reduction in the number of malaria cases leading up to the elimination of malaria in China, evidence-based control strategies, and relevant malaria prevention and control policies, have been synthesized before the formulation of control strategy. This way provided great evidence to formulate the National Malaria Control Programme and Malaria Elimination Programme. At the same time, a network of scientific research and surveillance has been established in China which produced a great number of expertise team in China. Through those activities, thousands of professional technical teams have been trained, and malaria control efforts within specific zones have been coordinated in the past six decades. By intensity interventions on surveillance and response, there has been a remarkable achievement since the early 1950s. By the late 1990s, the incidence of malaria significantly declined to tens of thousands from 2.4 million in 1970s, the endemic regions sharply shrunk, and *P. falciparum* malaria was eliminated in all regions except for Yunnan and Hainan Provinces. By 2009, the national total number of malaria cases was reduced to 14,000, and among 24 malaria endemic provinces, the malaria incidence in 95% of the counties dropped below 1/10,000 of incidence rate, with only 87 counties having more than 1/10,000. The data indicate that China has transited from malaria control to malaria elimination.

The importance of sharing experiences with other LMICs

The Chinese experience in terms of country-own and country-led efforts to combat the malaria epidemic is able to be tailored to Africa, where many countries have faced severe challenges in the control of the disease, partly due to limitations in public health systems as well as infrastructure. One of studies to compare the historical changes in malaria incidence between China and African countries indicated that, both China and Africa are located in the tropical and sub-tropics with optimal climatic and environmental conditions for the reproduction and development of *Anopheles* species. In the era of 1950s–1980s, the fluctuation patterns of malaria incidence were quite similar between China and African countries, while after 1980, the malaria incidence in China was declined significant and still keep the similar fluctuation patterns as before in Africa countries. The major reasons to appear the gap between Chinese and African incidence of malaria which become bigger are because of that although strengthening interventions has produced significant reduction of the malaria burden through nation-wide coverage of malaria control measures in some African countries, such as South Africa, Zanzibar, Gambia, Senegal, Ethiopia, Rwanda, Tanzania and Mozambique, the scaling up impact has not been the same in all African countries, such as The Democratic Republic of Congo (DRC) and Nigeria with a persistent burden of the disease (Figure 2.5).[6] Therefore, it was suggest to sustain the scaling up those interventions urgently in African countries especially learning from those have successfully health policies coupled with the sustained programmes in China. Furthermore, novel integrated control strategies aiming at moving malaria from epidemic status to control towards elimination, require solid research in understanding of the epidemiology, pathogenesis, vector dynamics, and socioeconomic aspects of the disease. Therefore, it is urgent for Chinese professionals to understand the importance of translating lessons learnt from the Chinese malaria control achievements and successes into practical interventions in malaria endemic countries in Africa and elsewhere, of which there were an estimated 216 million cases of malaria and 445,000 deaths worldwide, 90% of which occurred in Sub-Saharan Africa according to the 2017 World Malaria Report. Since China has been a major trading and investment partner of African countries, recently, the Chinese government has promised to continue increasing its support and investment in Africa, which includes medical assistance as well as the promotion of sustainable development. In July 2012, the former World Health Organization (WHO) Director-General Dr. Margaret Chan emphasized the importance of health cooperation between Africa and China during her visit to China, and the Chinese leader of the central government gave a positive response. While in the Beijing Declaration signed by both Chinese government and 53 African countries as well as several international agencies in 2013, malaria was one of 8 priorities in the agenda of the China-Africa health cooperation. Therefore, malaria control and elimination will be future priority work cooperated between China and African collaboration.

Pilot project in sharing Chinese experience on malaria control

A pilot project on malaria control was established in 2016 between China and Tanzania, since malaria epidemic in Tanzania is the number one cause of morbidity and

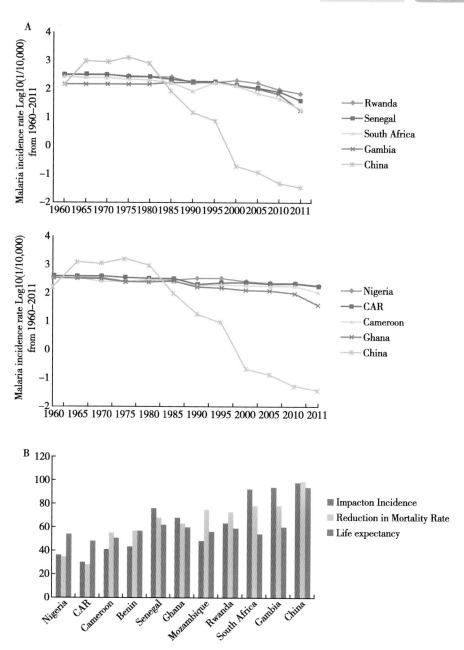

Figure 2.5 (A) Trend in malaria incidence rate Log₁₀ (1/10,000) in selected African countries and China from 1960–2011. (A1) Substantial scaling up impact on malaria incidence in China and some African countries; (A2) Scaling up impact on malaria incidence in China and low/moderate outcomes in some African countries). (B) Overall scaling up impact on incidence and mortality rate, and life expectancy in selected African countries and China in 2011. CAR, Central Africa Republic.

mortality among children aged below five years and adults as well. In order to share the knowledge and experiences on health system reforms across the two countries, and to test the feasibility of Chinese experiences implemented in local malaria situation of Tanzania in the form of China-Africa collaboration, a pilot project, namely "China-UK-Tanzania Pilot Project on Malaria Control", has been launched by supported by UK Department for International Development (DFID), was implemented by the National Institute of Parasitic Diseases (NIPD) at China CDC and Ifakara Health Institute (IHI) in Tanzania from April, 2015 to June, 2018, in 4 wards of Rufiji District in Tanzania, including two intervention communities and two control communities. By the end of June, 2018, the main findings of this pilot project were: (i) there were no malaria related deaths reported from the local health facilities in the intervention communities; (ii) the parasite prevalence were reduced by 81% (from 25.7% in 2015 to 4.9% in 2018) and by 52% (from 28.1% in 2015 to 13.4% in 2018) in the high and low intervention communities, respectively; (iii) an adapted new approach for malaria control was developed, that is a 1–7 malaria Reactive Community-based Testing and Response approach. This pilot project collaborated between China and Africa in the field of malaria control was the first step in strengthening cooperation and activities on public health between the two countries. The scaling up activities will be follow up to demonstrate the feasibility of Chinese experiences in malaria control in multi-regions of Africa which was supported by Bill & Melinda Gates Foundation (BMGF).

2.2.3　Action plan for transition from control to elimination of malaria in China

China intends to eliminate indigenous malaria nationwide by 2020, with the first step to find no indigenous cases outside of Yunnan province by 2015. With this goal in mind, China's malaria elimination plan was formulated with the following elements.

Case finding

Pilot testing of screening for glucose-6-phosphate dehydrogenase (G6PD) deficiency is ongoing. G6PD screening to be rolled out in all *P. vivax* endemic areas with a high prevalence of G6PD deficiency pending results of pilot tests.

Treatment

Focused mass drug administration "Spring treatment" program; 180 mg primaquine is administered over eight days to patients who had *P. vivax* in the year prior, to people who close contacts with positive *P. vivax* cases in the year prior, and occasionally to entire villagers. The efficacy of this program is currently under study.

Diagnosis

Strengthening diagnosis, treatment, and reporting are planned. All cases were diagnosed by microscopy or RDTs in the medical falcilities.

Surveillance

1-3-7 surveillance approach, based on the national web-based case reporting system, comprises case reporting within 24 hours, case verification and investigation within 3 days, and foci investigation and response to inhibit the secondary transmission within 7 days. All residents living in villages with at least one confirmed case are screened with microscopy and polymerase chain reaction (PCR). The global positioning system (GPS) is used to record the locations of the positive cases.

Entomological surveillance and vector

Indoor residual spraying is used at active foci with any malaria incidence. Vector species identification, density, and insecticide resistance are monitored at sentinel sites.

Control

High-risk populations are poor ethnic groups, forest workers, ethnic minority groups, highly mobile populations, and adult males (due to work and propensity to sleep outside without a bed net). Mobile medical teams are used to improve malaria treatment provided to migrant workers and local residents on the border areas. Targeted interventions planned to increase coverage of treatment among high-risk populations by 2015 include distributing malaria packs of long-lasting insecticide-treated nets (LLINs), prophylactic medications, and behavior change communication (BCC) materials to border crossers at the Yunnan-Myanmar border; providing BCC materials and extra LLINs for use overnight to Hainan forest workers; providing BCC materials through peer groups to Anhui migrant workers; modifying case management policy as appropriate after pilot screening tests to ethnic minority groups with a higher G6PD deficiency prevalence; and distributing LLINs through antenatal clinics to pregnant women and children.

Health education

Health education is administered in the form of BCC materials being provided to school students, and it needs to be strengthened. High-risk groups (forest workers, migrant workers) receive BCC materials from peer groups and non-governmental organizations. Chinese nationals who travel to endemic countries receive pre-departure information, text messages during the transmission season, and are screened and treated at airports upon return.

The goal of the health education program under NMEP was formulated as follows: by 2012, 75% of elementary and high school students should have knowledge of malaria prevention and treatment, and this figure should reach 85% by 2015. Finally, by 2020, awareness of malaria should be improved further and people should participate in malaria prevention, control, and elimination more proactively.

Challenges in the elimination of malaria

Although great achievements have been made in the transition from malaria control to elimination, the challenges for eliminating malaria in China need to be well understood. The major challenges are summarized below:

First, *Anopheles sinensis* is the primary vector of *P. vivax* in China, and climate change (i.e. increasing temperatures) may contribute to improving its efficiency of transmission and life span.

Second, populations at risk of malaria, including people who cross the Yunnan-Myanmar border, forest workers, and migrant workers, pose a challenge to the malaria elimination program, as they are often hard to reach. China's elimination strategy includes numerous plans to implement targeted delivery of health services and supplies to these at-risk groups.

Third, imported malaria cases are increasing and threatening to resurge malaria in China, particularly in the areas where proper species of mosquitoes existing. There are about 3,000 imported malaria cases presented annually in China. Mostly those who have come back from African or Asian countries are infected with various species of parasites, mostly *P. falciparum*, followed by *P. vivax, P. malariae*, and *P. ovale*.[7,8]

2.2.4　Conclusion

China has achieved remarkable successes to reach the goal of malaria transmission control and malaria elimination through the national malaria control programme before 2009 and NMEP after 2010, respectively. But, we are still facing multiple challenges to sustain the free malaria in the country. Those challenges are as follows: (i) inadequate and untimely information exchange on the status of imported malaria among different areas; (ii) inadequate collaborative action among malaria-endemic countries, especially around China-Myanmar border, which often do not provide relevant information to persons leaving their territory; (iii) surveillance information including epidemic data, resident population and floating population did not well managed and exchanged between the countries on a regular basis; (iv) Lack of close collaboration in monitoring susceptibility of malaria vectors to various insecticides as well as drug-resistant parasites in border areas; (v) lack of awareness of malaria reintroduction into areas free of malaria among the general health services staff; (vi) inadequacies in malaria training, particularly it is lack of collaboration in training activities among existing training centres and facilities in the regions; (vii) immature country-level partnership in malaria control, particularly it is still lack of mechanism in dealing with the imported *P. falciparum* malaria, in cooperated with more provinces in the malaria-free areas in China as well as other border countries.

　　In order to achieve the best possible preparedness for malaria reemerging, following activities need to be taken: (i) performing on potential risk assessment on malaria re-transmission in epidemic-prone areas are urgently to be conducted, such as risk districts or areas with an originally high malaria endemic potential, risk population moving from non- and low-endemic areas to highly malarious areas, and risk factors in changes of meteorological conditions; (ii) multi-sector cooperation between the health services and immigration and quarantine services, customs and police, which is very useful for acquiring information on the entry of possibly infected sources. Vigilance is necessary to step up at the airports and other ports which malaria cases pass through; (iii) implementing antianopheline measures in areas with high risk of transmission to prevent malaria resurgence; (iv) adequate briefings for travellers and the availability in the market of recommended antimalarials; and (v) providing more training in all hospitals and local authorities to improve the capability in case detection and diagnosis of malaria.

References

1. Zhou ZJ. The malaria situation in the People's Republic of China. Bull World Health Organ, 1981, 59(6): 931-936.

2. Wang RB, Zhang QF, Zheng B, et al. Transition from control to elimination: impact of the 10-year global fund project on malaria control and elimination in China. Adv Parasitol, 2014, 86: 289-318.

3. Yin JH, Yang MN, Zhou SS, et al. Changing malaria transmission and implications in China towards National Malaria Elimination Programme between 2010 and 2012. PLoS One, 2013, e74228.

4. Zhou XN, Xia ZG, Wang RB, et al. Feasibility and roadmap analysis for malaria elimination in China. Adv Parasitol, 2014, 86: 21-46.

5. Feng XY, Xia ZG, Vong S, et al. Surveillance and response to drive the national malaria elimination program. Adv Parasitol, 2014, 86: 81-108.

6. Tambo E, Adedeji AA, Huang F, et al. Scaling up impact of malaria control programmes: a tale of events in Sub-Saharan Africa and People's Republic of China. Infect Dis Poverty, 2012, 1(1): 7. doi: 10.1186/2049-9957-1-7.

7. Feng J, Xia ZG, Vong SD, et al. Preparedness for Malaria Resurgence in China: Case Study on Imported Cases in 2000–2012. Adv in Parasitol, 2014, 86: 231-65.

8. Qian YJ, Zhang L, Xia ZG, et al. Preparation for malaria resurgence in China: approach in risk assessment and rapid response. Adv Parasitol, 2014, 86: 267-88.

2.3 Application of spatial epidemiology in malaria control

2.3.1 Introduction

Malaria seriously impedes the socioeconomic development of developing countries, including China. After 40 years of dedicated efforts, the Chinese malaria control program has made great achievements. However, due to geographical, environmental, and social factors, malaria in the remaining transmission areas are difficult to control. Resurgence or even an outbreak of malaria may occur. It is thus imperative to use existing knowledge of biology, epidemiology, and new technologies to set up an early warning system that can predict and forecast the spread of the disease.

The transmission of malaria is determined by the existence of a causative agent, the host, and environmental factors. The disease transmission pattern is influenced by a certain time point, certain place, and certain population group. The occurrence, development, and elimination of a disease have specific regularity. A better under-standing of the distribution characteristics of a disease can guide the design and implementation of relevant control strategies.

The emergence and development of geographic information system (GIS) and remote sensing (RS) techniques have allowed new ways of detecting diseases and conducting environmental surveillance. These techniques are expected to become one of the routine monitoring tools for timely tracking, monitoring, and control of diseases. The GIS/RS provide a scientific basis for the allocation of limited resources and coordination between humans and their environment with the goal of improving human health. In the 21st century, the GIS/RS have been used in the monitoring of a variety of vector-borne diseases, e.g. schistosomiasis, malaria, filariasis, dengue fever, Lyme disease, etc. in Africa, South America, Asia, and other regions. In China, many researches have been conducted on the application of the GIS/RS on analysis of malaria transmission patterns.

Collecting spatial information helps to track changes in the living environment of malaria vectors. Thus, the application of GIS becomes a prerequisite for malaria control. In practice, GPS and RS technologies are usually combined. The GPS is a navigation system providing spatial and temporal information for all weather set-tings. Four or more GPS satellites without obstructed lines of sight orbiting the Earth receive this information. The system provides critical capabilities to military, civil, and commercial users around the world. Remote sensing allows for the archiving of information regarding an object or phenomenon without direct contact. The term usually denotes the use of aerial sensor technologies to distinguish objects via broad-casted signals (e.g. electromagnetic radiation). It may be split into passive (e.g. sun-light) or active (when a signal is first emitted from an aircraft or satellite) RS, when information is merely recorded.

Prevention and surveillance are both important components in malaria control programme. Surveillance is also important for measuring the malaria situation and evaluating the effects of implementation. The application of advanced technology in real-time, dynamic, and long-term monitoring can paint a complete picture of the abundance and distribution of malaria cases and analyze the transmission interruption situation in a timely manner, in order to determine the cause of the spread and thereby the scientific control strategy. The GIS, RS, and GPS (referred to collectively as the "3S") technologies are currently able to meet these demands. The GIS has the functions of data acquisition, storage, management, spatial analysis, display, and result output. For diseases with characteristics of temporal and spatial transmission patterns, the GIS can visualize epidemiological data, analyze spatial data, and construct epidemiological models. In addition, the GIS can provide new ways of determining how to allocate health resources, conduct regional health planning, and determine the spatial relationship between healthcare systems, disease distribution, and influence factors. Remote sensing is gradually being used in the prevention of parasitic diseases. It has many advantages, such as a large detection range, high updating frequency, ability to provide real-time information, and it is less subject to ground conditions. Some studies have been conducted on mosquito breeding site detection to prevent and control malaria. The GPS provides precise positioning and orientation, which can be used to identify the locations of positive cases or vector breeding sites. The use of combined 3S technology can make data access, updating, processing, and analyzing more accurate. Disease prevention, monitoring, forecasting, and control in the field can be entirely integrated. Thus, 3S technology provides a powerful tool for guiding malaria control activities in the field.

Recently, mathematical or statistical models have been applied to the study of disease transmission. They can quantitatively describe the impact of the etiology, host, and environment on disease transmission using mathematical equations. Practice in the field then feedbacks to evaluate and modify the models. Therefore, it is important to use modern mathematical methods to analyze the distribution and transmission pattern of infectious diseases in order to establish an epidemiological model for prevention and control.

2.3.2   Spatial technology in the monitoring and prediction of malaria

In the prevention and control of malaria, Centers for Disease Control and Prevention (CDCs) at all levels in China usually take response actions after a malaria outbreak or epidemic takes place. There are difficulties in using traditional methods to predict or forecast disease transmission accurately, which may in turn cause a serious loss of resources and people's lives. Due to the spread of drug-resistant malaria, combined with frequent domestic and international population movement, malaria control is getting more difficult. As the spread of malaria is related to specific environmental and epidemiological factors, predicting or forecasting malaria transmission can be possible with surveillance response systems. Recently, with the development and application of public health information theory and technology, such as 3S techniques, predicting the malaria endemic situation via the establishment of surveillance response systems is looking possible. At least three areas have been applied in China as described below:

Predicting the malaria transmission season and intensity

Tian[1] applied GIS techniques and extracted malaria transmission-associated climatic factors to create a multiple regression model in order to predict malaria incidence. Out of the investigated climatic factors, it was found that humidity was the dominant factor affecting malaria transmission. The study also found that introduced comprehensive climate—environmental factors—soil moisture had more advantages than rainfall. This model can be applied in similar settings at the macro level to quantitatively predict the impact of global warming on local malaria transmission.

Using GIS, Zhang et al. [2] established a national malaria epidemic geographic information database and analyzed the characteristics of malaria incidence trends and temporal distribution between 2006 and 2010. The study indicated that the incidence of malaria during these five years showed an overall decreasing trend. The peak of malaria incidence was between July and October each year. Through spatial and temporal analysis, the malaria transmission pattern could be identified, thus determining malaria control focal areas.

Wen et al. [3] collected data on monthly malaria incidence, monthly temperature, monthly rainfall, and monthly relative humidity in each Hainan municipality, and also extracted the average monthly vegetation index, the maximum monthly vegetation index, and the minimum monthly vegetation index from AVHRR satellite images. A multivariate regression model was then developed to explore the relationship between malaria prevalence and the natural environment in Hainan. It was found that rainfall during the rainy season (May to October) influences the malaria epidemic as it affects the amount of vegetation. The population density of mosquitoes is closely related to rainfall and thus indirectly affects the intensity of malaria transmission.

Yang et al. [4] combined environmental factors with the GIS to establish a biology-driven model that meets the effective surveillance response needs of malaria transmission in China. Environmental data of 676 locations in China were collected, and smoothed surface maps showing the number of months suitable for parasite survival were generated based on monthly mean temperature and yearly relative humidity. The study showed that malaria transmission regions had shifted northwards over the past few decades, which was confirmed in practice.

Xiao et al. [5] used spatial and temporal quantitative methods to explore the relationship between the incidence of malaria and climate factors. The spatial distribution of malaria was mapped using the cumulative and annual malaria incidence rates of each county. The temporal trends of malaria were calculated using the Cochran-Armitage trend test. It was found that the average temperature of the previous few months in an area can be used to predict the incidence of malaria.

Zhang et al. [6] adopted the GIS and time-series analysis to explore the risk factors of malaria transmission, while also examining the spatial and temporal heterogeneities of malaria. The study showed a strong seasonal pattern, with the highest malaria incidence from July to November. In terms of spatial distribution, the annual malaria incidence was found to spread from the north to the south. The study concluded that the yearly average temperature is an important factor influencing malaria incidence. It was concluded that the application of the GIS would benefit the optimization of malaria surveillance in China.

Yang et al. [7] established a malaria prediction model based on the parasite growing degree day, which predicted malaria endemic areas and transmission intensity in

Jiangsu Province. Meteorological data of the province and its surrounding areas were extracted from the World Meteorological Organization's FAOCLIM. The total growing degree days (TGDDs) were calculated and mapped using ArcView 3.0a software. The TGDD malaria prediction map showed that the malaria epidemic gradually reduced from the west to the east in Jiangsu, and was divided into three zones, which was consistent with the map showing the average malaria incidence over the past 14 years.

Wang et al. [8] established a malaria GIS database based on county-level malaria surveillance data between 1990 and 2006 in Anhui Province. Spatial scanned cluster analysis using SaTScan™ software detected three hot spots in the province. First-level clustering areas were in the northern region in 2004–2006, mid-western region in 1990–1992, and mid-eastern region in 1990–1991, which indicated that the epidemic was moving north.

Predicting the spatial distribution of malaria transmission

Zeng et al. [9] investigated malaria distribution patterns in different geographical environments. A database with information on land use, altitude, and malaria epidemics in Hainan Province using the GIS/RS was established, and then thematic maps were produced. The results showed that the central and southern regions dominated by forest coverage had a higher incidence of malaria. The study suggests that the transmission trend and intensity of malaria can be predicted based on the type of coverage.

Yang et al. [10] predicted malaria distribution and spread trends by applying satellite RS data, and generated a national map showing malaria endemic areas. Meteorological data from the National Weather Station and malaria incidence data from monitoring sites were collected. Yearly averaged NDVI images derived from NOAA-AVHRR satellite data were processed using the ERDAS IMAGINE 8.x software platform. NDVI values from the National Weather Station and of malaria surveillance points were extracted, which were used for correlation analysis and prediction of malaria endemic regions. It was determined that the NDVI was positively correlated with rainfall and relative humidity, of their R^2 were 0.3018 and 0.2565, respectively. In addition, it was found that NDVI values in malaria endemic areas were >140, which was applied to predict the national malaria transmission rate.

Yang et al. [11] generated a surface smoothed map showing malaria parasite temperative growing degree days (TGDDs), rainfall, and relative humidity using ArcView 3.0a software. Delphi expert consulting results indicated that the contribution of the aforementioned three environmental factors to malaria transmission was 5:3:2, which was consistent with previous results reported in literature. A multi-layer map was produced by overlaying the maps of TGDDs, rainfall, and relative humidity with the weight of 5:3:2.

Su et al. [12] established a Hainan malaria incidence GIS database and created a malaria spatial distribution map by spatial local interpolation analysis in ArcGIS 8.1 software. It was concluded that the spatial local interpolation method can correctly estimate the spatial distribution of malaria in Hainan, and thereby guide the implementation of appropriate control measures.

Zhang et al. [13] used malaria monitoring incidence data between 1978 and 1999 in Jiangsu Province to produce a malaria transmission smoothed map, which showed that the high-risk areas were in Xuhuai Plain and the low-risk areas were in Taihu Lake region.

Gao et al. [14] created malaria incidence thematic maps based on 1997–2001 malaria incidence and mortality data in provinces, municipalities, and autonomous regions of China using MapInfo Professional 5.5 software. The results showed a high incidence rate in Yunnan and Hainan Provinces. July to September was found to be the peak time interval of malaria incidence.

Zhou et al. [15] established a malaria incidence GIS database of 156 counties in the Huang-Huai River region in 2005 using ArcGIS software. A smoothed surface map of malaria indicated the spread or diffusion trend of malaria to surrounding areas. malaria incidence showed a significant spatial clustering in the Huang-Huai River basin.

Predicting vector habitats and monitor the vector population

Three major environmental factors, namely temperature, humidity, and rainfall, impact mosquito reproduction and life span.

Temperature also affects malaria parasite development within mosquitoes. Generally, temperatures lower than 16 or higher than 30 degrees are not conducive to *An. sinensis* mosquito development and can inhibit the proliferation rate of *Plasmodium* sporozoites. The lowest temperature for developing *P. vivax* in *An. sinensis* mosquitoes is 14.5 degrees, which restricts the malaria endemic regions. Regions with altitudes higher than 3,000 meters are malaria free due to low temperatures.

There is no direct effect of relative humidity on the malaria parasite, however, it does influence the activities and life span of the vector. Low relative humidity shortens the life span of the mosquito. If the monthly average relative humidity is less than 60%, there is no malaria transmission.

Rainfall affects malaria transmission in a complex way. Rainfall not only changes the temperature, but also increases the relative humidity, and often expands vector breeding sites. In some areas, flooding can cause malaria outbreaks, while in others drought causes outbreaks. The rainy season always determines the malaria transmission season of the year. In lowland waterlogging areas of temperate regions, the malaria peak season is always after the rainy season, while in tropical rainforest areas, the malaria peak season is before the rainy season. Understanding the ecology of the vector can help to develop appropriate countermeasures, thus suppressing the number of mosquitoes to a low level in order to halt the spread of malaria. On the other hand, mosquito breeding sites and numbers can be predicted based on changes in environmental factors, and thus indirectly predict malaria epidemics.

Anopheles mosquitos are the main vectors of malaria transmission, spreading the pathogens between people. The breeding sites and reproduction of *Anopheles* are closely related to environmental factors. Factors that affect malaria are numerous, complex, and diverse. Characteristics of mosquito breeding sites, density of larvae and adult mosquitoes, and their relationship with the environment need to be explored intensively to improve prediction accuracy.

El-Zeiny et al. [16] collected information on mosquito breeding sites using the GPS and extracted highly quantified environmental data from RS images. The associations between mosquito population density and related factors were analyzed. Using RS overcomes shortcomings when doing ecological studies on a large scale, such as time-consuming, laborious, and non-visualized. High-resolution satellite data also provide a convenient way to investigate the relationship between mosquitoes and the environment at the micro level.

Zhou et al. [17] recognized the association between malaria cases and distribution of water bodies by spatial analysis, in order to provide guidance for effective strategies formulation based on highlighted at-risk populations and areas. The malaria case data (357 malaria cases) and case-related GPS data, as well as nearby water bodies data were assembled and analyzed. It was found that 74% of malaria cases were situated in the 60-meter buffer zone adjacent to the water bodies. The risk ratio of people having malaria and living close to water bodies was significantly higher than that of others (OR = 1.6, 95%CI = 1.042, 2.463, $P < 0.05$).

Ren et al. [18] investigated malaria data from 62 sentinel surveillance sites in China between 2005 and 2008. Linear mixed effects models were applied to detect the major ecological factors of *An. sinensis* human biting rates (HBIs) and the spatiotemporal variation of related factors at the surveillance sites. A low *A. sinensis* HBI was associated with an increasing distance to the nearest river ($\beta = -1.47$ [-2.88, -0.06]), while a higher *An. sinensis* HBI was significantly associate with the minimum semimonthly temperature ($\beta = 2.99$ [2.07–3.92]), enhanced vegetation index ($\beta = 1.07$ [0.11–2.03]), and paddy index (the percentage of rice paddy fields in the total cultivated land area) ($\beta = 0.86$ [0.17–1.56]). The temporal variation ($\sigma(s0)(2) = 0.83$) of biting rates was larger than the spatial effect ($\sigma(t)(2) = 1.35$).

Liu et al.[19] used the GIS to analyze the relationship between the population density of *An. sinensis* and *An. jeyporiensis* mosquitoes, and environmental factors in the southern region of Yunnan Province. The following geographical factors were determined: paddy field areas within one kilometer distance buffer from the light, river length within one kilometer distance buffer from the light, distance from light to the nearest river, and distance from light to the nearest rice fields. A multiple linear regression model was constructed to show the associations between mosquito population density and the aforementioned four geographical factors. It was found that the closer the distance was to the rice fields, the higher the *A. sinensis* density was and the lower the *An. jeyporiensis* density was.

2.3.3   Challenges with and prospects of spatial technology in malaria control research

Spatial technology is able to monitor temporal and spatial distribution of malaria in real-time and dynamically, determining the potential habitats of *Anopheles* mosquitoes and predicting malaria transmission. It provides a strong technical support for in-depth malaria control and possesses the advantages with which traditional technology and methods are incomparable. However, there are still many problems in the practical application of 3S technology for malaria control. The three main ones are: (i) RS images, spectra, radiation, and temporal resolution need to be improved as mosquito breeding habitats in small water bodies cannot be accurately identified; (ii) resource-based GIS data, such as basic topographic data, population resources, meteorological resources, health information and other resources belonging to different departments, are difficult to share in epidemiological studies, it is difficult to access the latest RS images and other related environmental information in a timely manner; the cost of the data is relatively expensive and the data structure is not uniform, which thus limits the data's application in the health field; and (iii) spatial techniques applied in malaria control are multidisciplinary, involving medicine, geography, computer science, biology, and other subjects. Capacity building is thus a priority issue.

In addition, with in-depth research on malaria transmission being conducted, comprehensive factors apart from environmental factors, such as sociodemographic characteristics, urbanization, population growth, and changes to vectors need to be considered and introduced into models to improve their accuracy. Although GIS/RS technology has gradually become an effective tool in malaria research, it does not mean this technology can replace conventional surveillance methods. It is recommended that spatial analysis techniques and traditional onsite investigations are combined to fully understand the impacts of natural and social factors related to malaria in order to achieve the goal of better prevention and control of the disease, and contribute to its early warning.

Due to the powerful spatial analysis capabilities of the GIS technology, and with the launch of high-resolution satellites; continuous improvement of computer hardware, and GIS and RS software; GPS accuracy; as well as the development and application of web GIS, spatial technology will play a massive role in malaria control in the following areas: (i) surveillance and monitoring; (ii) management and resource allocation; (iii) forecasting and modeling; (iv) establishment of intelligent GIS; and (v) the development of malaria information systems. With the establishment of a malaria spatial database, formation of spatial thinking, and improvement in sharing consciousness of collaboration, the epidemiology of malaria is experiencing a tremendous change.

2.3.4   Conclusion

It is well known that malaria is a life-threatening disease caused by parasites transmitted to humans through the bites of infected mosquitoes. Malaria is on the list of category B notifiable infection diseases to be reported as according to the Law of Communicable Diseases Prevention and Control of China. The facts are that (i) malaria is transmitted by female *Anopheles* mosquitoes, (ii) there are over 15 species of *Anopheles* mosquitoes in the Western Pacific Region capable of malaria transmission, with each having its own breeding preferences and biting habits; and (iii) malaria is preventable and curable, with the key interventions including prompt and effective treatment with artemisinin-based combination therapies (ACTs), use of insecticidal nets by people at risk, and indoor residual spraying with insecticides to control the vectors. Artemisinin-resistant *P. falciparum* malaria remains one of the biggest challenges in malaria control and elimination in the Great Mekong sub-region (GMS). While containment efforts on the Cambodia-Thailand border have been successful, new foci of resistance are being discovered in other areas, necessitating a regional containment strategy. Therefore, all aforementioned factors need to be considered and related to surveillance response systems in the design of protocols for national malaria elimination.

Summary fact box

- In China, endemic malaria is caused by two types of parasites, namely *P. falciparum* and *P. vivax*.
- Reported malaria cases have declined dramatically in China through years of efforts. The annual incidence of malaria was reduced to tens of thousands by the end of the 1990s from 24 million at the beginning of the 1970s.
- In 2010, the Chinese government launched a national campaign on malaria elimination, with the goal of eliminating the disease throughout China by 2020.

- In 2011, 1,398 *P. falciparum* malaria cases were reported in 28 provinces, of which, 1,366 were imported. Among the imported cases, 1,111 were reported in 26 non-*P. falciparum* malaria endemic provinces.

- In 2011, the number of cases of imported *P. falciparum* malaria in non-endemic provinces increased by 49.13%, with 30 deaths, which was double the number in 2010.

- The epidemic area of *P. falciparum* malaria in China has been significantly narrowed to Yunnan and Hainan Provinces in the late of 2000s.

- According to national guidelines, the treatment for *P. falciparum* malaria is ACTs, while chloroquine plus primaquine is still used for treating *P. vivax* malaria.

- China has been working on a therapeutic efficacy study of antimalarial drugs in Yunnan Province since 2008, supported by the WHO. To date, there is no evidence of confirmed artemisinin resistance in China.

References

1. Tian LW, Bi Y, Ho SC, et al. One-year delayed effect of fog on malaria transmission: a time-series analysis in the rain forest area of Mengla County, south-west China. Malar J, 2008; 7: 110

2. Zhang Y, Liu QY, Luan RS, et al. Spatial-temporal analysis of malaria and the effect of environmental factors on its incidence in Yongcheng, China, 2006–2010. BMC Public Health, 2012, 12(1): 544.

3. Wen L, XU DZ, Wang SQ, et al. Epidemic of malaria in Hainan Province and modeling malaria incidence with meteorological parameters. Chin J Dis Control Prev, 2003, 7 (6): 520-524. (in Chinese)

4. Yang G, Tanner M, Utzinger J, et al. Malaria surveillance-response strategies in different transmission zones of the People's Republic of China: preparing for climate change. Malaria J, 2012, 11(1): 426.

5. Xiao D, Long Y, Wang S, et al. Spatiotemporal distribution of malaria and the association between its epidemic and climate factors in Hainan, China. Malaria J, 2010, 9(1): 185.

6. Zhang Y, Liu QY, Luan RS, et al. Spatial-temporal analysis of malaria and the effect of environmental factors on its incidence in Yongcheng, China, 2006-2010. BMC Public Health, 2012, 12(1): 544.

7. Yang G, Zhou X, Malone JB, et al. GIS prediction model of malaria transmission in Jiangsu Province. Chin J Prev Med, 2002, 36(2): 103-105. (in Chinese)

8. Wang LP, Xu YF, Wang JJ, et al. Spatial-temporal analysis on the distribution of malaria in Anhui, 1990-2006. Chin J Dis Control Prev, 2008, 12 (2): 156-159. (in Chinese)

9. Zen X, Ye S, Xu C, et al. Correlation of malaria epidemic situation in Hainan Province by remote sensing and geographic information. J Third Mili Med Univ, 2015, 37(8): 821-826. (in Chinese)

10. Yang GJ, Gao Q, Zhou SS, et al. Mapping and predicting malaria transmission in the People's Republic of China, using integrated biology-driven and statistical models.. Geospat Health, 2010, 5(1): 11-22.

11. Yang G, Zhou X, JB Malone, et al. GIS prediction model of malaria transmission in Jiangsu Province. Zhouhua Yu Fang Yi Xue Za Zhi, 2002, 36(2): 103-105. (in Chinese)

12. Su YQ, Zhang ZY, Xu DZ. Application of remote sensing and GIS technology in malaria epidemiological study. People's Military Surgeon, 2005, 48(9): 540-542. (in Chinese)

13. Zhang XP, Jin XL, Yang GJ, et al. Spatial analysis on transmission tendency of malaria based on surveillance data in Jiangsu. Chin J Zoonoses, 2002, 18(1): 120-121. (in Chinese)

14. Gao CY, Xiong HY, Han GH, et al. Prevalence and characteristics of malaria in China. J Third Mili Med Univ, 2003, 25(11): 974-976. (in Chinese)

15. Zhou SS, Huang F, Tang LH, et al. Study on the spatial distribution of malaria in Yellow River and Huai River areas based on the Kriging method. J Pathogen Biol, 2007, 2(3): 204-206. (in Chinese)

16. El-Zeiny A, El-Hefni A, Sowilem M. Geospatial techniques for environmental modeling of mosquito breeding habitats at Suez Canal Zone, Egypt. Egypt J Remote Sensing Space Sci, 2017, 20(2): 283-293.

17. Zhou SS, Zhang SS, Wang JJ, et al. Spatial correlation between malaria cases and water-bodies in Anopheles sinensis, dominated areas of Huang-Huai Plain, China. Parasit Vectors, 2012, 5(1): 106.

18. Ren Z, Wang D, Hwang J, et al. Spatial-temporal variation and primary ecological drivers of Anopheles sinensis human biting rates in malaria epidemic-prone regions of China. PLoS One, 2015, 10(1): e0116932.

19. Liu MD, Wang XZ, Zhao TY, et al. Geographic information system analysis on the relationship of populations of Anopheles sinensis and An. jeyporiensis with the environment factors in Yunnan Province. Chin J Vector Biol Control, 2008, 19(4): 275-279. (in Chinese)

2.4　New tools for detecting low-density malaria in elimination settings

The continuously shrinking malaria map takes us one step closer towards world-wide eradication of malaria. However, numerous challenges still exist. To eliminate malaria and prevent resurgence, the surveillance response system must be able to detect all possible malaria infections in the area in a timely manner to effectively interrupt transmission.[1] In low endemic areas, targeted active case detection (ACD) is the most widely adopted surveillance approach, whereby either all high-risk individuals at the community level or passively detected cases are screened for infection and treated with rapid response measures, including radical treatment and targeted vector control.[2, 3] Since 2010, China has implemented a highly successful "1-3-7" ACD surveillance approach: one day to report a case, three days to confirm and classify a case, and seven days to conduct local response and prevent any onward transmission.[2] While these operational measures are effective against outbreaks, their positive impact on elimination remains to be demonstrated.

2.4.1　Diagnostics: The key to malaria elimination

The accuracy of malaria diagnosis is essential for the effectiveness of elimination measures. Microscopy and rapid diagnostic tests (RDTs) are the diagnostic methods implemented in most elimination programs, both of which are recommended by the WHO.[4, 5] While the sensitivities of these methods are generally sufficient to diagnose acute malaria cases, they have significant limitations in settings where the infection rate is low, as a substantial proportion of cases might not show any symptoms, the parasite density is lower than the threshold needed for detection by microscopy or RDT, and they have been estimated to result in 20–50% of all transmission episodes.[6] A recent trial of large-scale community-wide screening using RDT in Burkina Faso found no impact of ACD on parasite prevalence or incidence of clinical episodes after 12 months of follow-up.[7] This was most likely due to the poor sensitivity of the RDT to detect all parasitemic and gametocytemic individuals.[7]

　　Molecular methods, such as polymerase chain reaction (PCR),[8] quantitative real-time PCR,[9] nucleic acid sequence-based amplification (NASBA),[10] and loop-mediated isothermal amplification (LAMP) [11] have better sensitivity, yet their dependence on nucleic acid purification significantly influences their diagnostic performance.[9–11] They are also labor-intensive in surveillance settings when dealing with large numbers of samples. Importantly, the target amplification nature of these methods is prone to contamination, which leads to false-positive results, restricting their application to laboratories with specially trained technicians and sophisticated equipment.[12]

Most molecular assays target DNA of the *Plasmodium* multicopy 18S rRNA genes[8, 9] due to their high copy numbers (4–8 copies per parasite[13]) and mosaics of conserved and variable regions, which is ideal for both genus and species identification. Besides the 18S rRNA gene, many other high-copy genes have recently been reported as an equivalent/better diagnostic target, including the telomere-associated repetitive element 2 (TARE-2, ~250 copies/genome) and the var gene acidic terminal sequence (varATS, 59 copies/genome).[14] Targeting expressed nucleic acid sequence (RNA), rather than the gene itself, has been increasingly considered in recent years for better sensitivity.[15–22] A-type 18S rRNA genes, for example, are stably expressed at 1×10^4 copies per ring-stage parasite,[18] which is logs more abundant than that of the gene. This increase in concentration of the target significantly improves sensitivity of assays and thereby enables accurate identification of asymptomatic, subpatent infections.[18, 19] However, most RNA-based tests are highly demanding on facilities and techniques due to their reliance on RNA purification and reverse transcription. The lability of RNA compared with the durability of DNA also discourages these assays for clinical use.[22]

As malaria control programs approaching elimination, an increasing number of case tests have to be performed in order to find one positive infection. This was the case in 2013 in Yunnan Province, when more than 350,000 cases were screened to find 460 infections. To encourage community-wide participation, the WHO proposed that all active screening services be free of charge.[23] Increased massive screenings placed an elevated burden on a surveillance system that was already challenged by a heavy workload and limited funding. These challenges necessitated the innovation of technology for malaria elimination, calling for tests with a higher throughput and lower cost, in addition to being highly sensitive, which is a requirement for detecting asymptomatic infections. This has been accepted as one of the top priorities in the field.[6]

There are at least three adverse consequences for malaria elimination that have to be immediately addressed. Firstly, a lack of accurate diagnostic tests and precise estimates of community prevalence results in clinicians often ignoring negative test results, and overprescription of antimalarial drugs is common.[24] In some low prevalence areas, less than 1% of patients treated with an antimalarial drug had malaria parasites in their blood.[25] This overdiagnosis of malaria at healthcare facilities coexists with an underdiagnosis of malaria in the community, with the result that sometimes antimalarials are given to healthy individuals and not given to sick ones.[26] More effective, and also more expensive, drugs, such as ACTs, have to be introduced to control or eliminate the disease.[27] However, high levels of misdiagnosis[28] are not cost effective and may give rise to drug resistance.

Secondly, without reliable active population screening, malaria surveillance programs that measure only clinical illness will not give an accurate estimation of the prevalence of parasitemia and probability of infection as countries head for elimination.[29, 30] This will result in unreliable modeling of risks, cost effectiveness, and feasibility of eliminating and maintaining elimination, ultimately affecting the commitment to the elimination policy.[31–33]

Finally, with no effective high throughput (HTP) assay to screen large numbers of at-risk travelers and migrants, most of whom show no symptoms, malaria can easily resurge.[12] It is therefore evident that sensitive and HTP diagnostic tests play an essential part in malaria elimination programs.

2.4.2　Two novel diagnostic assays: RNA hybridization assay and capture and ligation probe-PCR (CLIP-PCR)

Chinese researchers have developed two novel HTP molecular assays for malaria: sandwich RNA hybridization assay with branched DNA technology[17] and CLIP-PCR[15]. Both methods simplified the "sample to result" procedure into an enzyme-linked immunosorbent assay (ELISA)-like process, significantly reducing test complexity and labor demand.

The sandwich RNA hybridization assay with branched DNA technology quantifies RNA in a 96-well plate format without the need for RNA purification, reverse transcription, and target amplification. It is performed with a series of oligonucleotide probes containing target-specific sequences and probes containing an additional "tail" sequence that is independent of the target sequences, but can interact with either the solid support or the detection system. These probes are called capture extenders (CEs) and label extenders (LEs), respectively. The probes bind a contiguous or near-contiguous region of the target RNA. The CEs bind to the capture oligonucleotides conjugated to the surface of each well in a 96-well plate and, via cooperative hybridization, capture the associated target RNA. Signal amplification is mediated by DNA amplification molecules that hybridize to the tails of the LEs, and DNA amplification molecules can then be detected by a chemiluminescent reaction (Figure 2.6).[34]

The limit of detection (LoD) was determined as the minimal amount of erythrocyte-cultured P. falciparum added to the erythrocytes that gave a net signal three

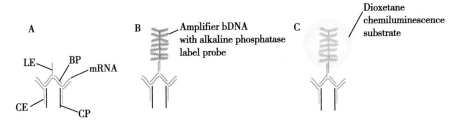

Figure 2.6   The sandwich RNA hybridization assay process. (A) For each RNA target, a set of oligonucleotide probes capable of hybridizing a contiguous region of the target RNA molecule is designed. Some of these probes contain a common extension "tail" sequence that is independent of the target sequence but can interact with the solid support. These probes are called CEs. Other probes, called LEs, contain a different common tail sequence that can interact with the detection system. The remaining probes containing only target-specific sequences are called blockers (BLs). After samples are lysed and the released RNAs hybridize with their probes, multiple RNA-bound CE tails hybridize to the complementary capture probes (CPs) covalently attached to the solid support, leading to the capture of RNA to the solid support. (B) A bDNA molecule (20) is then applied and hybridized to the tails of the LEs. The branches of the molecule hybridize to oligonucleotide probes labeled with alkaline phosphatase. (C) Chemiluminescence detection is used to measure signals generated from the labeled probes after luminescent substrate dioxetane is added. The solid support is the surface of each well of a 96-well plate.

times higher than the SD of the background erythrocyte control. The sandwich RNA hybridization assay gave a detection limit of about 0.04 parasite/μL, which is above the threshold proportional to parasite numbers ($R^2 = 0.999$) (Figure 2.7).

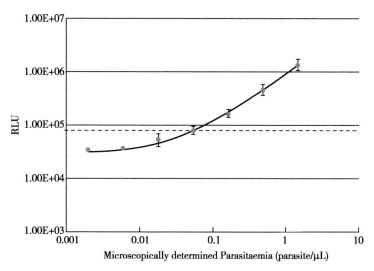

Figure 2.7 Correlation of assay signal with cultured *P. falciparum* parasitemia in human erythrocytes. Parasitemia in human erythrocyte culture was determined. The LoD was determined as the minimal amount of cultured *Plasmodium* added to the erythrocytes that gave a net signal three times higher than the SD of the background erythrocyte control (shown as a dotted line). Each dilution was prepared using a culture medium. Triplicate samples were used in the assay and the data are representative of three independent runs. The average LoD was 0.04 parasite/μL blood. RLU, relative light unit.

In a screen of 202 febrile patients from malaria endemic areas, the results in sandwich RNA hybridization assay was compared with that of microscopy, RDT, and genus-specific real-time PCR. As shown in Table 2.2, the assay detected three false-negative microscopy results and four false-negative RDT results, and was 100% in agreement with the real-time PCR diagnosis. No negative sample as detected by the RNA hybridization assay showed up positive using the other methods. This suggests that the RNA hybridization assay is at least as sensitive and specific as standard real-time PCR.

The 18S rRNA from dried blood spots (DBSs) was also tested. The stability of RNA in DBSs was determined by spotting cultured *P. falciparum* (50 parasites/μL) in 75-μL aliquots onto Whatman™ 903 filter paper, storing it with a desiccant at room temperature, 4°C, or –20°C, and then testing. No significant differences were observed in the results for up to 12 days of storage (Figure 2.8).

Table 2.2   Comparison of microscopy, RDT, standard real-time PCR, and RNA hybridization assay.

		RNA hybridization assay (*n* = 202)	
		Positive (n = 69)	*Negative (n = 133)*
Microscopy (*n* = 202)	Positive	66 (27 P.f + 39 P.v)	0
	Negative	3	133
RDT (*n* = 143)	Positive	6	0
	Negative	4	133
Standard real-time PCR (*n* = 152)	Positive	19	0
	Negative	0	133

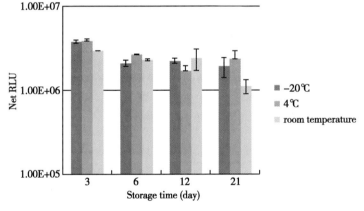

Figure 2.8   Stability of RNA in DBSs.

In a similar process, CLIP-PCR quantifies 18S rRNA of the genus *Plasmodium* by the amount of ligated probes that bind continuously to it (Figure 2.9).

The analytical LoD was determined to be 0.01 parasite/μL for the 3D7 parasite strain (Figure 2.10). To increase the assay throughput and reduce per-sample assay cost, the ability of CLIP-PCR to detect target RNA in pooled DBSs was evaluated. Pooling of positive DBSs with negative ones did not significantly reduce the detection signal (Figure 2.11) and a pool size of more than 20 made it difficult to pipette enough lysate for duplicate tests. A second elution of large pools produced

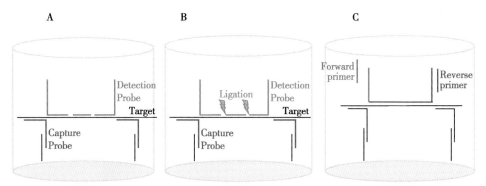

Figure 2.9   CLIP-PCR process. (A) During overnight incubation of a sample lysate, CPs (including two regions, one for target binding and the other for anchoring the target) and detection probes (DPs) bind to a contiguous part of a highly conserved region in *Plasmodium* 18S rRNA; the CP anchors the target to solid surface by hybridizing with probes on the solid surface. (B) After the unbound probes are washed off, DPs, which bind adjacent to each other, are ligated to form a longer ssDNA. The DPs located at both ends also include an extra region as a universal primer binding site. (C) The newly ligated ssDNA, the quantity of which is proportional to the target RNA, is quantified by real-time PCR with a universal primer set and SYBR® Green chemistry.

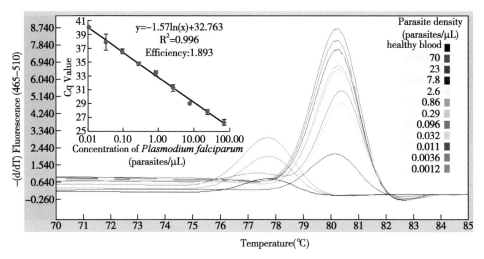

Figure 2.10   The analytical LoD determined as 0.01 parasite/μL for the 3D7 parasite strain. A 3-fold, 11-point serial dilution of *P. falciparum* (strain 3D7) was made in whole blood lysate. The concentration ranged from 70 p/μL to 0.0012 p/μL, with each tested twice by CLIP-PCR. Cq values from duplicate tests were plotted against concentration. Samples with concentrations lower than 0.01 are deemed as negative by melting curve analysis, and are therefore not included in the plot.

only a reduced signal (see Figure 2.11). Although centrifugation retrieves lysate more effectively, this procedure adds complexity, which may give rise to cross-contamination.

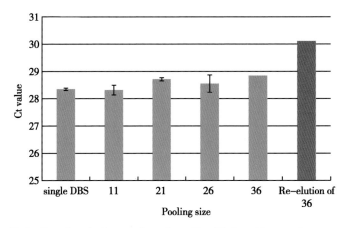

Figure 2.11 Detection signal after pooling of positive DBSs with negative ones. DBSs were prepared by spotting 75-µL cultured *P. falciparum* strain 3D7 (50 parasites/µL) or whole blood from healthy volunteers to Whatman™ 3MM filter paper and air-dried for four hours. A single positive DBS (50 parasites/µL) was mixed with 0, 10, 20, 25, or 36 negative DBSs separately, and tested as a single sample by CLIP-PCR. Duplicate testing was applied to a pool of 26 or less, while lysate of pool size 36 was only sufficient for one test; the residue was eluted again with a 100 µL lysis mixture for the second test.

As pooling of less than 26 DBSs exerts little influence on the signal produced by the positive one, the pooling strategy can therefore be conducted in large-scale screening to save time, labor, and cost, while maintaining efficiency. There are several pooling strategies that can be considered, among which matrix-based pooling (Figure 2.12) [15] and hierarchical pooling (Figure 2.13) [35] are the two most popular ones. In matrix-based pooling, each sample is tested twice in different contexts, and is therefore less prone to false-negative results. In addition, as the positive signal directly indicates the coordinate of the positive sample, this pooling strategy does the job in a single run if each matrix contains no more than one positive sample. This can be very efficient when screening for low prevalence infections. However, matrix-based pooling requires more labor than hierarchical pooling, especially in endemic settings where the positive rate is high. Therefore, the hierarchical pooling strategy should be considered in settings where the percentage of positive cases might be higher than 2–4%.

In an active screening of malaria in 3,358 DBS samples, the CLIP-PCR method was coupled with matrix-based pooling. It finished the screening with less than 500 tests (each test done twice), identifying 14 infections (Table 2.3).

Table 2.3   Active screening of 3,358 DBS samples.

Sample No.	Mean Cq values* of CLIP-PCR (SD*)	Mean Cq values* of standard real-time PCR (SD*)	Clinical symptom(s) on sampling day	RDT	Microscopy
9	–	–	None	+	–
61	–	–	None	+	–
67	–	–	None	+	–
69	31.0 (0.02)	31.1 (0.17)	None[a]	–	–
80	33.9 (1.02)	34.1 (0.28)	None[b]	–	–
117	35.1 (0.81)	35.0 (0.10)	None[c]	–	–
208	34.1 (0.67)	34.5 (0.24)	None[d]	–	–
LD572	24.4 (0.20)	29.2 (0.06)	Fever	N/A	+
LD508	23.9 (0.21)	31.6 (0.07)	Fever	N/A	+
LD519	28.4 (0.12)	33.5 (0.03)	Fever	N/A	+
LD518	22.6 (0.43)	32.0 (0.06)	Fever	N/A	+
LD575	23.9 (0.17)	30.1 (0.03)	Fever	N/A	+
LD649	21.3 (0.28)	31.9 (0.14)	Fever	N/A	+
LD617	23.2 (0.20)	31.0 (0.06)	Fever	N/A	+
LD652	21.6 (0.44)	30.0 (0.04)	Fever	N/A	+
2–210	30.0 (N/A)	31.1 (0.29)	Fever	N/A	+
2–8	26.7 (0.05)	34.1 (0.05)	Fever	N/A	+

*Mean values and standard deviations (SDs) are calculated from results of duplicate tests.

N/A: not tested/not applicable; +: positive; –: negative; a, b, c, and d: the patient developed a malaria-related syndrome after sampling within two months, 10 days, one month, and two weeks, respectively. For standard real-time PCR, the first seven patients in this study were tested using whole blood samples, while others were tested using DBS samples.

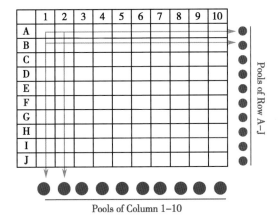

Figure 2.12 Matrix pooling process. Samples in the same row are pooled and tested together as one, and so are the samples in the same column. The figure shows an example of a 10 × 10 matrix in which, sample C5, for example, is tested once in the tube containing Pool C and once in the tube containing Pool 5. All 100 samples are analyzed twice by testing Pool A to J and Pool 1 to 10 (a total of 20 tests).

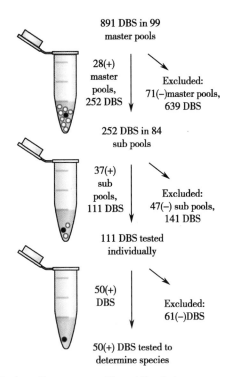

Figure 2.13 Hierarchical pooling process. The white circles represent *Plasmodium*-negative DBSs; the black circles represent *Plasmodium*-positive DBSs. At each stage, the DBSs were tested as one sample.

2.4.3　The right diagnostics in the right settings

Both the RNA hybridization assay and CLIP-PCR can directly detect 18S rRNA in whole blood/DBS samples in a 96-well plate format with comparable sensitivity and specificity to standard real-time PCR, while eliminating the reliance on RNA purification and reverse transcription. As their processes and performances are identical, the differences between the two assays for end users are the machine that reads the plate and the format of test results. As results of both assays are essentially self-explanatory, users could make the selection according to what machine they have in the laboratory.

These two RNA screening assays enable large-scale screening of tens of thousands of people. In such scenarios, it is difficult to perform one-by-one rapid, field-friendly diagnostic tests. A model involving centralized, highly parallel laboratory testing that is quality-assured and involves adequately trained personnel makes more sense, as it saves resources and time while ensuring high-quality results.

Given the definitive status of microscopy and the unsurpassed ease of use and rapid diagnosis time of RDTs, it is not expected that molecular assays will replace microscopy or RDTs for routine clinical diagnosis. Instead, these assays can complement these tests, for example, for quality assurance in clinical settings or to screen large numbers of at-risk population samples for accurate, rapid, and cost-effective assessment of community prevalence. Perhaps the combination of quality-assured RDT/microscopy diagnosis in health facilities and the practice of regular active community surveys at the district level will provide the needed assurance to clinicians to prescribe drugs in alignment with malaria test results, resolving the current issue of malaria overdiagnosis in many low transmission areas.

As very low levels of transmission are reached, malaria programs will move from a focus on control to a focus on pre-elimination and elimination, and finally prevention of malaria reintroduction. Molecular assays become very attractive when used for active malaria monitoring, evaluation, and surveillance; for accurate evaluation of transmission in near-eliminated areas; or for screening large numbers of travelers and migrants to prevent reintroduction. A two-tiered approach is proposed: first, screening for infections among large numbers of samples with RNA hybridization assay or CLIP-PCR, and then testing the positive samples using current available methods such as real-time PCR for confirmation and species identification. While molecular assays cannot be used as "field-ready" as RDTs, they should be deployable in a district laboratory with services that provide ELISA-type tests and should be able to be handled by technicians with little training beyond standard routine clinical laboratory practices.

References

1. Liu J, Modrek S, Gosling RD, et al. Malaria eradication: is it possible? Is it worth it? Should we do it? Lancet Global Health, 2013; 1(1): e2-e3.

2. Cao J, Sturrock HJW, Cotter C, et al. Communicating and Monitoring Surveillance and Response Activities for Malaria Elimination: China's "1-3-7" Strategy. PLoS Med, 2014, 11(5): e1001642.

3. Sturrock HJW, Hsiang MS, Cohen JM, et al. Targeting Asymptomatic Malaria Infections: Active Surveillance in Control and Elimination. Plos Med, 2013; 10(6): e1001467.

4. World Health Organization. World malaria report: 2013. 2014.

5. World Health Organization. Guide lines for the treatment of malaria, Second edition. 2010. http://whqlibdoc.who.int/publications/2010/9789241547925_eng.pdf (Accessed Jun 18, 2014).

6. Cotter C, Sturrock HJ, Hsiang MS, et al. The changing epidemiology of malaria elimination: new strategies for new challenges. Lancet, 2013, 382(9895): 900-11.

7. Tiono AB, Ouedraogo A, Ogutu B, et al. A controlled, parallel, cluster-randomized trial of community-wide screening and treatment of asymptomatic carriers of Plasmodium falciparum in Burkina Faso. Malar J, 2013, 12: 79.

8. Snounou G, Viriyakosol S, Jarra W, et al. Identification of the four human malaria parasite species in field samples by the polymerase chain reaction and detection of a high prevalence of mixed infections. Mol Biochem Parasitol, 1993, 58(2): 283-92.

9. Rougemont M, Van Saanen M, Sahli R, et al. Detection of four Plasmodium species in blood from humans by 18S rRNA gene subunit-based and species-specific real-time PCR assays. J

Clin Microbiol, 2004, 42(12): 5636-43.

10. Mens PF, Schoone GJ, Kager PA, et al. Detection and identification of human Plasmodium species with real-time quantitative nucleic acid sequence-based amplification. Malar J, 2006, 5: 80.

11. Lucchi NW, Demas A, Narayanan J, et al. Real-Time Fluorescence Loop Mediated Isothermal Amplification for the Diagnosis of Malaria. PLoS One, 2010, 5(10): e13733.

12. The malERA Consultative Group on Monitoring E, and Surveillance. A research agenda for malaria eradication: diagnoses and diagnostics. PLoS Med, 2011, 8(1): e1000396.

13. Mercereau-Puijalon O, Barale JC, Bischoff E. Three multigene families in *Plasmodium* parasites: facts and questions. Int J Parasitol, 2002, 32(11): 1323-44.

14. Hofmann N, Mwingira F, Shekalaghe S, et al. Ultra-sensitive detection of *Plasmodium falciparum* by amplification of multi-copy subtelomeric targets. PLoS Med, 2015, 12(3): e1001788.

15. Cheng Z, Wang D, Tian X, et al. Capture and ligation probe-PCR (CLIP-PCR) for molecular screening, with application to active malaria surveillance for elimination. Clin Chem, 2015, 61(6): 821-8.

16. Xiaodong S, Tambo E, Chun W, et al. Diagnostic performance of CareStart malaria HRP2/pLDH (Pf/pan) combo test versus standard microscopy on falciparum and vivax malaria between China-Myanmar endemic borders. Malar J, 2013, 12: 6.

17. Cheng Z, Sun X, Yang Y, et al. A novel, sensitive assay for high-throughput molecular detection of plasmodia for active screening of malaria for elimination. J Clin Microbiol, 2013, 51(1): 125-30.

18. Murphy SC, Prentice JL, Williamson K, et al. Real-time quantitative reverse transcription PCR for monitoring of blood-stage *Plasmodium falciparum* infections in malaria human challenge trials. Am J Trop Med Hyg, 2012, 86(3): 383-94.

19. Taylor BJ, Martin KA, Arango E, et al. Real-time PCR detection of *Plasmodium* directly from whole blood and filter paper samples. Malar J, 2011, 10: 244.

20. Kamau E, Tolbert LS, Kortepeter L, et al. Development of a highly sensitive genus-specific quantitative reverse transcriptase real-time PCR assay for detection and quantitation of plasmodium by amplifying RNA and DNA of the 18S rRNA genes. J Clin Microbiol, 2011, 49(8): 2946-53.

21. Adams M, Joshi SN, Mbambo G, et al. An ultrasensitive reverse transcription polymerase

chain reaction assay to detect asymptomatic low-density *Plasmodium falciparum* and *Plasmodium vivax* infections in small volume blood samples. Malar J, 2015, 14(1): 520.

22. Zimmerman PA, Howes RE. Malaria diagnosis for malaria elimination. Curr Opin Infect Dis, 2015, 28(5): 446-54.

23. WHO. Disease Surveillance for malaria elimination: An operational manual. 2012.

24. Sansom C. Overprescribing of antimalarials. Lancet Infect Dis, 2009, 9(10): 596.

25. Reyburn H, Mbakilwa H, Mwangi R, et al. Rapid diagnostic tests compared with malaria microscopy for guiding outpatient treatment of febrile illness in Tanzania: randomised trial. BMJ, 2007, 334(7590): 403.

26. Ansah EK, Narh-Bana S, Epokor M, et al. Rapid testing for malaria in settings where microscopy is available and peripheral clinics where only presumptive treatment is available: a randomised controlled trial in Ghana. BMJ, 2010, 340: c930.

27. Ogutu B, Tiono AB, Makanga M, et al. Treatment of asymptomatic carriers with artemether-lumefantrine: an opportunity to reduce the burden of malaria? Malar J, 2010, 9: 30.

28. Lubell Y, Reyburn H, Mbakilwa H, et al. The impact of response to the results of diagnostic tests for malaria: cost-benefit analysis. BMJ, 2008, 336(7637): 202-5.

29. Cibulskis RE, Aregawi M, Williams R, et al. Worldwide incidence of malaria in 2009: estimates, time trends, and a critique of methods. PLoS Med, 2011, 8(12): e1001142.

30. Harris I, Sharrock WW, Bain LM, et al. A large proportion of asymptomatic *Plasmodium* infections with low and sub-microscopic parasite densities in the low transmission setting of Temotu Province, Solomon Islands: challenges for malaria diagnostics in an elimination setting. Malar J, 2010, 9: 254.

31. Feachem RG, Phillips AA, Targett GA, et al. Call to action: priorities for malaria elimination. Lancet, 2010, 376(9752): 1517-21.

32. Alonso PL, Brown G, Arevalo-Herrera M, et al. A research agenda to underpin malaria eradication. PLoS Med, 2011, 8(1): e1000406.

33. The malERA Consultative Group on Monitoring E, and Surveillance. A research agenda for malaria eradication: monitoring, evaluation, and surveillance. PLoS Med, 2011, 8(1): e1000400.

34. Zheng Z, Luo Y, McMaster GK. Sensitive and quantitative measurement of gene expression directly from a small amount of whole blood. Clin Chem 2006, 52(7): 1294-302.

35. Hsiang MS, Lin M, Dokomajilar C, et al. PCR-based pooling of dried blood spots for detection of malaria parasites: optimization and application to a cohort of Ugandan children. J Clin Microbiol, 2010, 48(10): 3539-43.

Chapter 3

Immunoproteomic Platform for Antigen Screening of Human Parasitic Infections for Serodiagnostic and Vaccine Development

Kassegne Kokouvi and Jun-hu Chen

3.1 Introduction

Biomarkers for serodiagnostics and vaccine development for malaria and neglected tropical diseases (NTDs) have been hampered by the limited availability of antigens identified using the so-called "traditional" techniques such as two dimensional chromatography, mass spectrometry, reverse immunogenetics, etc. Although these approaches have been applied to screen immunoreactive proteins, and have been useful in the identification of candidate antigens and proteins profiling in a high throughput (HTP) manner, they are inappropriate for assessing HTP antibody profiling and are also inadequate to efficiently identify large amounts of promising candidate targets.[1-4] Therefore, substantial improvements are needed to accelerate the identification of efficient candidate antigens that target parasite-specific stages for vaccine pipelines and serodiagnostics.

This chapter describes the capacity of an immunoproteomic approach that the National Institute of Parasitic Diseases (NIPD), Chinese Center for Disease Control and Prevention (China CDC) has developed as one of the promising tools for the identification of candidate antigens to effectively help control and eliminate human parasitic diseases. Rapid access to omics databases, state-of-the-art facilities, experiences in establishing an antigen screening platform, and strong testing and evaluation networks of current antigens are some of the advantages that make the NIPD, China CDC an ideal organization to build an innovative research and development platform.

This chapter summarizes the features of this approach that make it a powerful and innovative technology for antigen screening, and also provides an overview of antigen screening of human parasites using protein arrays. Moreover, the route and workflow of the platform developed at the NIPD are described. Lastly, the chapter highlights some of the pioneering efforts to actively translate antigen discoveries into controlling and eliminating parasitic diseases, as well as successful examples of international cooperation.

3.2 Protein arrays: cutting-edge technology for antigen screening

Defined as the reactivity of antigens with antiserum from parasite-exposed animals or individuals, protein arrays sense the magnitude of antibody responses to proteins regardless of the abundance of the antibody. Highly immunogenic proteins are further assessed as putative vaccines, while antigens for diagnosis are selected by comparing their immunoreactivity to serum samples from case-control cohorts. Thus, this technology has allowed for the exploration and analysis of both natural and induced humoral immune responses to several human parasites, and efficiently enables HTP antibody profiling for the identification of large amounts of candidate antigens that the so-called "traditional" approaches were not able to achieve. A large repertoire of human parasite antigens identified using protein arrays was described in a previous study.[2] The effectiveness of the platform relies on the following: (i) unique methodology for construction; (ii) time-efficient and cost-effective technique; and (iii) unique platform to rapidly profile large numbers of variant-specific humoral responses to infections. Moreover, the technology has been proven to be an excellent application of the genome of human pathogens as it provides a better understanding of parasite-host interactions and host immune responses.[5, 6] The approach has completely revolutionized research on vaccine epitopes and has improved the development of serodiagnostics for parasitic diseases that burden humans.

3.3 Antigen screening of human parasites using protein arrays

3.3.1 Introduction

In the last 10 years, antigen screening of human parasites using protein arrays has emerged as a powerful tool for antigen discovery, and its effectiveness is unquestionable. The PubMed database was searched for research articles on antigen screening of human parasites/parasitic diseases that used protein arrays. After excluding unrelated references and reviews or comments, a list of 60 articles was retained from January 2006 to July 2018. The results showed that, in terms of this technology, malaria has been the most intensively investigated among human parasitic infections, followed by schistosomiasis (Figure 3.1).[4, 11, 14] In addition, nearly 70% of the studies were carried out in the past three years, and antigen screening was performed to detect blood-stage target candidate antigens for the development of vaccines or serodiagnostic tests for malaria and NTDs.

3.3.2 Insights from global antigen screening studies

With respect to the studies conducted worldwide, protein arrays have provided general information about receptor-ligand interactions, and have been helpful in profiling clear antibody responses and identifying blood-stage immunodominant antigens. Comprehensively, investigations on malaria have profiled natural or induced antigen-specific antibody responses and anti-disease/sterile protective immunity,[4, 7, 8] and have also identified disease clinical protection in asymptomatic and naturally acquired immunity individuals, which were both associated with blood-stage antigen candidates for *P. falciparum* and *P. vivax*.[8-10] Other studies have validated and newly identified serological biosignatures using sera of individuals from malaria endemic areas.[6, 11] Recently, studies have showed that natural protective antibody responses against naive and semi-naive individuals experimentally challenged with *P. falciparum* sporozoites were associated with new candidate targets.[12] In addition, investigations carried out in the Peruvian Amazon showed that *P. falciparum* blood-stage proteins are

174

highly immunodominant and clinically immune when screened with infected asymptomatic individual sera.[9]

In terms of NTDs, schistosomiasis has been a major focus of investigations. The technology has importantly contributed to validating antigens and discovering potential novel targets. Areas of research have included: (i) natural or induced antibody profiles from infected hosts, and antibody signatures and disease pathologies in *Schistosoma japonicum*-infected individuals;[13,14] (ii) identification of antibody signatures and antigenic candidates for serodiagnostic and vaccine development to *S. mansoni*;[15] and (iii) identification of novel vaccine candidates through sera profiles of humans/primates resistant to *S. haematobium*. [16] Although antigen screening investigations for other NTDs have not been as pronounced as for schistosomiasis, the technique has also been applied to explore antigenic and immunogenic targets through antibody profiling using different types of infected sera to *Toxoplasma gondii*,[17, 18] *Trypanosoma cruzi*,[19, 20] *Babesia microti*,[21] *Echinococcus* spp. [22] *Necator americanus*,[5] and *Onchocerca volvulus*.[23] These findings constitute the basis for sensitive and specific serodiagnostic evaluation, as well as for candidate epitopes for vaccine development.

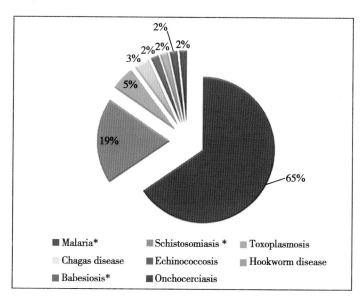

Figure 3.1   Percentage distribution of publications on antigen screening of human parasitic infections using protein arrays, from January 2006 to July 2018. (Data search up to July 2018.) *Antigen screening for parasitic diseases performed at the NIPD, China CDC.

3.3.3 Valuable input of the antigen screening approach developed at the NIPD

The NIPD has developed a platform for antigen screening which has contributed more than ever to the scientific knowledge of identified target candidates. Skillfully established about half a decade ago, the platform aims to acutely discover antigens of human parasites (Table 3.1). For example, in the studies carried out by Chen et al., a total of 169 highly immunoreactive *P. vivax* blood-stage antigens were identified, of which 12 were well-characterized vaccine candidates from previous studies, while the remaining 157 were new discoveries.[4, 6] Along similar lines, the same authors have profiled natural antibody responses to *P. falciparum* antigens and identified 30 highly immunogenic merozoite antigens, including ten blood-stage vaccine candidates which were previously identified. Additionally, seven protein targets and two hypothetical proteins were firstly reported to be immunogenic.[11] Importantly, among the seven *P. falciparum* antigen candidates discovered, the antigen epitope of *P. falciparum* thirty-four protein (Pf34) is highly immunogenic and thus considered as a novel promising vaccine candidate for *P. falciparum* malaria. Previously identified leading vaccine candidates for malaria such as *P. falciparum* circumsporozoite protein (PfCSP), *P. falciparum* apical membrane antigen 1 (PfAMA1), and *P. falciparum* merozoite surface proteins 1 and 3 (PfMSP1 and PfMSP3), to name a few, as well as the *P. vivax* circumsporozoite protein (PvCSP) have been validated.

Studies on the immunologoic analysis of the proteome of the parasites responsi-

Table 3.1 Studies carried out at the NIPD, China CDC on human parasite antigen screening using HTP protein arrays.

Diseases	Parasites	Study areas	References
Malaria	*P. falciparum*	Natural antigen-specific antibody profiles to *P. falciparum* blood-stage antigen	11
	P. vivax	Genome-level analysis of natural antibody responses to *P. vivax* infection	4
Schistosomiasis	*S. japonicum*	Natural antibody analysis of the tegument proteins of the human blood fluke	14
Babesiosis	*B. microti*	Explorative biomarkers screening using different types of infected sera	24

ble for NTDs have essentially been focusing on *S. japonicum*. The prominent investigation has been on *S. japonicum* tegument proteins, in which 30 highly immunoreactive tegument antigens were reported for the first time, of which the antigen epitopes of triosephosphate isomerase of *S. japonicum* Chinese strain (Sjc-TPI) is a leading vaccine candidate.[14] Protein arrays have also been applied to *B. microti* and a panel of potential antigens have been identified (unpublished data). In addition to these, it is noteworthy that current protein array-based investigations are being conducted to explore candidate antigens against other parasitic diseases that burden humans.

3.4   The route and workflow of the platform designed at the NIPD

3.4.1   Introduction

This section summarizes the workflow of the antigen screening platform developed at the NIPD. The procedure involves six important steps as described elsewhere[1, 2] and outlined (Figure 3.2).

3.4.2   Sampling of infected individual sera

The sources of antisera that are used to profile antigen-specific antibodies are of great importance in order to provide a better understanding of pathogen-host interactions and subsequent host immune responses. Thus, infected individual sera used to probe proteins are obtained from case-control studies, cross-sectional studies, and longitudinal cohort studies.

3.4.3   *In silico* data mining: selection of open reading frames (ORFs)

The release of genomic sequence data and transcriptome of many human parasites have boosted postgenomic research, radically linking genomics to proteomics. Thus, putative immunogenic targets of specific blood-stage parasites are selected from the genome using comparative genomics and immunoinformatics. The main selection criteria for ORFs are the presence of signal peptide and/or transmembrane domain(s) in the protein/peptide sequences.

3.4.4   Polymerase chain reaction (PCR) amplification of ORFs and HTP gene cloning

Selected ORFs are subsequently amplified using in-fusion primers, according to which each forward and reverse gene-specific primers are converted by extension at their 5' terminus in order to obtain PCR products that have linear ends with homology arms of the vector. Thereafter, the pEU recombinant vector is constructed using a HTP in-fusion gene cloning technique.

3.4.5   Wheat germ cell-free (WGCF) protein expression and detection of his-tagged protein

The WGCF protein expression technology is known for being a unique HTP protein expression system for overcoming challenges in antigen screening of human parasitic infections, especially as it has the capacity to efficiently synthesize, with high speed and precision, large amounts of proteins from genes that contain large number of A/T sequences. Explicitly, proteins are HTP expressed in a cell-free *in vitro* bilayer transcription–translation system using a highly purified recombinant plasmid. The expression level and the immunoreactivity of crude proteins are then analyzed.

3.4.6   HTP protein probing and antibody profiling

Protein probing and serum screening constitute the two main components of the antigen screening platform. Briefly, crude WGCF recombinant proteins, as well as positive and negative controls, are spotted as probes in duplicate on an array-specific slide and then incubated. Then, serum samples from parasite-specific exposed versus unexposed individuals are used to screen the probes. Bound antibodies are visualized using Alexa Fluor® 546 Goat Anti-Human Immunoglobulin G (IgG) and scanned in a fluorescent microarray scanner.

3.4.7   Bioinformatic approach to immunoproteomics

Antibody profiles to probed antigens are evaluated using the fixed circle approach to quantify the arrays. The two-tailed unpaired method is used to analyze the correlation between duplicate spots, antibody reactivity, and immune responses, and correct for false discovery rate. Thus, antigen candidates are assessed by comparing different cohorts of exposed and unexposed serum samples, or infection-resistant and -susceptible host groups.

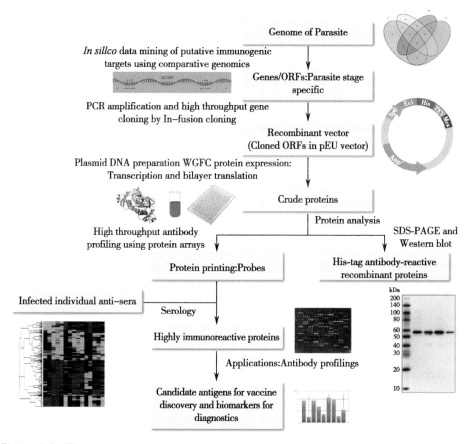

Figure 3.2   The route and workflow of the antigen screening approach designed at the NIPD, China CDC.

3.5 Applications of the HTP antigen screening platform

The fundamental application of HTP antigen screening is to identify candidate antigens for serodiagnostics and vaccine development, regarded as one of the promising strategies to accelerate the control and elimination of human parasitic diseases. In this regard, after candidate targets are identified, they are evaluated for sensitivity

179

and specificity through a combined blood screening strategy for serological markers or preclinical assessments for vaccine epitopes. The evaluation and validation tests not only guide the sensitivity and specificity of target candidates, but also aid in prioritizing suitable biomarkers for the development of diagnostics; firstly, detection of IgG antibodies using a large repertoire of infected individual sera through antigen-based assays (i.e. enzyme-linked immunosorbent assay, dipsticks, etc.), and secondly, comparison with standard methods (e.g. Kato-Katz stool examination for *Schistosoma* compared to a new diagnostic technique, and microscopic examination of blood smears compared to a new *Plasmodium* diagnostic method). For example, regarding a serological marker, studies carried at the NIPD have revealed the sensitivity and specificity of the *P. vivax* merozoite surface protein 1 (PvMSP1) to be 92.2% and 95.6%, respectively (unpublished). Implicitly, this and other highly sensitive and specific serodiagnostic antigens are currently being processed for the development of user-friendly IgG antibody detection kits for use in control and elimination programs, especially to monitor disease transmission in areas that are in the elimination stage. The sensitivity and specificity of potential diagnostic targets for other parasites are currently being studied, whereas preclinical evaluation of vaccine antigens/epitopes are yet to be conducted. In addition, candidate targets that are identified can be directly used for serodiagnosis or rapid screening of patients suspected of infection with NTDs via the convenient and versatile HTP protein arrays platform. In other words, the platform can improve the development of serodiagnostic tests, the evaluation of disease progression, and epidemiological research.[2] Recently, Chen et al. have successfully adapted the platform for massive screening of foodborne helminthiases.[25]

3.6 International cooperation to enable diagnostic development

Some key factors have contributed to the NIPD, China CDC, build a valuable service network for international cooperation. These include: strong capacity in the diagnosis and monitoring of human parasitic infections; experiences in designing an antigen screening platform; and pioneering efforts for strong testing and evaluation to actively translate antigens currently being discovered into the control and elimination of parasitic diseases.

The first collaborative project in the network is the World Health Organization (WHO) Demonstration Project entitled "Development for Easy to Use and Affordable Biomarkers as Diagnostics for Types II and III Diseases". This is a collaborative project between the African Network for Drugs and Diagnostics Innovation and (ANDI) partner institutions in Africa and the NIPD, as well as the China Network for Drugs and Diagnostics Innovation (China NDI). Through this project, open innovation, technology transfer, capacity-building, and South-South collaboration in support of sensitive, specific, and affordable diagnostic developments for NTDs in Africa are facilitated.[1] In this context, a successful training workshop has been implemented for young African and Chinese scientists from participating institutions and fellows from collaborating institutions, such as the Kenya Medical Research Institute in Kenya; the University of Health and Allied Sciences in Ho, Ghana; and the Theodor Bilharz Research Institute in Egypt. The participants were intensively trained for four weeks, from 5th to 30th September 2016, with an emphasis on knowledge transfer and capacity-building through practical training and theoretical courses on techniques/methods for diagnostic development for tropical diseases.

Another important project is the Australia-China-Papua New Guinea Pilot Cooperation on Malaria Control, a three-year project that commenced implementation in early 2016. The overarching objective is to contribute to reducing malaria morbidity and mortality in Papua New Guinea (PNG) through effective trilateral cooperation. To this end, the project has potentially planned some PNG- and China-based study design and analysis inputs to build/strengthen the capacity of research/public health personnel of PNG's key institutions in the areas of diagnosis and treatment of malaria. Thus, five representatives from three different PNG institutions (the Central Public Health Laboratory, the School of Medicine and Health Sciences of the University of PNG, and the PNG Institute of Medical Research), in partnership with the National Department of Health of PNG, have completed a study tour at the NIPD, China CDC. The participants were intensively trained for three weeks on molecular diagnostics, which intended to leverage their capacity to contribute to reducing malaria morbidity and mortality in PNG. The training essentially covered lectures, training courses, laboratory practical demonstrations, and round table discussions.

3.7 Conclusion

The application of the HTP antigen screening platform is one the strategies currently being used to accelerate the control and elimination of human parasitic diseases in China and worldwide. The fundamental objective of the platform is to identify candidate antigens for serodiagnostics and vaccines, and improve the development of serodiagnostic tests in the evaluation of disease progression and epidemiological research. This approach can effectively screen thousands of antigens simultaneously, identify their humoral responses, and profile the antibodies repertoire with meaningful statistical analysis that cannot be achieved using traditional approaches. At the NIPD, several successes have been recorded in the extensive application of the NIPD-developed platform to target parasite antigens. Hence, a large repertoire of human parasite candidate targets have been uncovered including species of *P. falciparum*, *P. vivax*, *S. japonicum*, and *B. microti*. Among these, some potential antigens/epitopes have been successfully assessed as serodiagnostics, whereas many others are currently being investigated for serological purposes and vaccine development pipelines.

References

1. Kassegne K, Zhang T, Chen SB, et al. Study roadmap for high-throughput development of easy to use and affordable biomarkers as diagnostics for tropical diseases: a focus on malaria and schistosomiasis. Infect Dis Poverty, 2017, 6(1): 130.

2. Kassegne K, Abe EM, Chen JH, Zhou XN. Immunomic approaches for antigen discovery of human parasites. Expert Rev Proteomics, 2016, 13(12): 1091-1101.

3. Chen SB, Ai L, Hu W, et al. New anti-*schistosoma* approaches in the People's Republic of China: development of diagnostics, vaccines and other new techniques belonging to the 'Omics' Group. Adv Parasitol, 2016, 92: 385-408.

4. Chen JH, Chen SB, Wang Y, et al. An immunomics approach for the analysis of natural antibody responses to *Plasmodium vivax* infection. Mol Biosyst, 2015, 11(8): 2354-63.

5. Tang YT, Gao X, Rosa BA, et al. Genome of the human hookworm Necator americanus. Nat Genet, 2014, 46(3): 261-9.

6. Chen JH, Jung JW, Wang Y, et al. Immunoproteomics profiling of blood stage *Plasmodium vivax* infection by high-throughput screening assays. J Proteome Res, 2010, 9(12): 6479-89.

7. Baum E, Sattabongkot J, Sirichaisinthop J, et al. Common asymptomatic and submicroscopic malaria infections in Western Thailand revealed in longitudinal molecular and serological studies: a challenge to malaria elimination. Malar J, 2016, 15: 333.

8. Finney OC, Danziger SA, Molina DM, et al. Predicting antidisease immunity using proteome arrays and sera from children naturally exposed to malaria. Mol Cell Proteomics, 2014, 13(10): 2646-60.

9. Torres KJ, Castrillon CE, Moss EL, et al. Genome-level determination of *Plasmodium falciparum* blood-stage targets of malarial clinical immunity in the Peruvian Amazon. J Infect Dis, 2015, 211(8): 1342-51.

10. Crompton PD, Kayala MA, Traore B, et al. A prospective analysis of the Ab response to *Plasmodium falciparum* before and after a malaria season by protein microarray. Proc Natl Acad Sci U S A, 2010, 107(15): 6958-63.

11. Fan YT, Wang Y, Ju C, et al. Systematic analysis of natural antibody responses to *P. falciparum merozoite* antigens by protein arrays. J Proteomics. 2013; 78: 148-58.

12. Arevalo-Herrera M, Lopez-Perez M, Dotsey E, et al. Antibody profiling in naive and semi-immune individuals experimentally challenged with *Plasmodium vivax* sporozoites. PLoS Negl Trop Dis. 2016; 10(3): e0004563.

13. Driguez P, Li Y, Gaze S, et al. Antibody signatures reflect different disease pathologies in patients with schistosomiasis due to *Schistosoma japonicum*. J Infect Dis. 2016; 213(1): 122-30.

14. Chen JH, Zhang T, Ju C, et al. An integrated immunoproteomics and bioinformatics approach for the analysis of *Schistosoma japonicum* tegument proteins. J Proteomics. 2014; 98: 289-99.

15. Gaze S, Driguez P, Pearson MS, et al. An immunomics approach to schistosome antigen discovery: antibody signatures of naturally resistant and chronically infected individuals from endemic areas. PLoS Pathog. 2014; 10(3): e1004033.

16. Pearson MS, Becker L, Driguez P, et al. Of monkeys and men: immunomic profiling of sera from humans and non-human primates resistant to schistosomiasis reveals novel potential vaccine candidates. Front Immunol. 2015; 6: 213.

17. Felgner J, Juarez S, Hung C, et al. Identification of Toxoplasma gondii antigens associated with

different types of infection by serum antibody profiling. Parasitology. 2015; 142(6): 827-38.

18. Liang L, Doskaya M, Juarez S, et al. Identification of potential serodiagnostic and subunit vaccine antigens by antibody profiling of toxoplasmosis cases in Turkey. Mol Cell Proteomics. 2011; 10(7): M110 006916.

19. Durante IM, La Spina PE, Carmona SJ, et al. High-resolution profiling of linear B-cell epitopes from mucin-associated surface proteins (MASPs) of *Trypanosoma cruzi* during human infections. PLoS Negl Trop Dis. 2017; 11(9): e0005986.

20. Carmona SJ, Nielsen M, Schafer-Nielsen C, et al. Towards high-throughput immunomics for infectious diseases: use of next-generation peptide microarrays for rapid discovery and mapping of antigenic determinants. Mol Cell Proteomics. 2015; 14(7): 1871-84.

21. Cornillot E, Dassouli A, Pachikara N, et al. A targeted immunomic approach identifies diagnostic antigens in the human pathogen *Babesia microti*. Transfusion. 2016; 56(8): 2085-99.

22. List C, Qi W, Maag E, et al. Serodiagnosis of *Echinococcus* spp. infection: explorative selection of diagnostic antigens by peptide microarray. PLoS Negl Trop Dis. 2010; 4(8): e771.

23. Lagatie O, Van Dorst B, Stuyver LJ. Identification of three immunodominant motifs with atypical isotype profile scattered over the *Onchocerca volvulus* proteome. PLoS Negl Trop Dis. 2017; 11(1): e0005330.

24. Zhou X, Huang JL, Shen HM, et al. Immunomics analysis of *Babesia microti* protein markers by high-throughput screening assay. Ticks Tick Borne Dis. 2018.

25. Chen JX, Chen MX, Ai L, et al. A protein microarray for the rapid screening of patients suspected of infection with various food-borne helminthiases. PLoS Negl Trop Dis. 2012; 6(11): e1899.

Chapter 4

Drug Development in China

Hao-bing Zhang and Qi Zheng

4.1 Introduction

Development of drugs to treat malaria and neglected tropical diseases (NTDs) has been one of the research priorities in China since the beginning of the National Control Program on Parasitic Diseases. In the 1950s, all research institutes of parasitic diseases established a group of professionals for the screening and development of new antiparasitic drugs, as no effective drugs existed for treating parasitic diseases.

4.2 Antimalarial drugs

In the early 1960s, chloroquine resistance in *Plasmodium falciparum* parasites was detected in Southeast Asia. Following this, drug-resistant strains continued to spread quickly throughout Asia, the Americas, Oceania, and many areas of Africa. Drug resistance was also found in Hainan, Yunnan, and Guangxi Provinces in China. In the late 1960s, the Chinese government carried out nationwide antimalarial drug research through the establishment of animal models, and synthesized new structures, as well as the screening of active structures which were extracted from traditional Chinese medicine. Great progress has been made, with research groups having developed many new antimalarial drugs such as artemisinin, hydroxypiperaquine phosphate, pyronaridine, its analogues pyracrine phosphate, and nitroquine. Among these new drugs, artemisinin and pyronaridine are the two main clinical medications. The new antimalarial drugs mostly originated from a national collaborative project named the "Mission 523" for screening new antimalarial drugs.

The Science and Technology Commission of the People's Republic of China and the People's Liberation Army's General Logistics Department held a national meeting on malaria prevention, treatment, and drug research collaboration on May 23, 1967. It urged for the development of new drugs to treat drug resistance of *P. falciparum* malaria in tropical areas, long-term prevention drugs, and anophelifuge. As this was a military project, it was known as "Mission 523" for confidentiality purposes. More than 60 scientific research units and 500 technical personnel participated in this project.

The "Mission 523" developed a detailed three-year research plan, with its missions divided into five main topics: (i) chemical synthesis and screening of new drugs for malaria prevention and control; (ii) traditional Chinese medicine and acupuncture for malaria control; (iii) development of anophelifuge; (iv) malaria drug formulation and packaging research; and (v) evaluating the effect of antimalarial drugs in the field.[1]

4.2.1 Development of an animal model for antimalarial drugs

Before developing new drugs, the "Mission 523" imported two types of rodent malaria (*P. berghei* NK65 and *P. yoelii*) and three types of simian malaria (*P. cynomolgi*, *P. inui*, and *P. knowlesi*). Then, four types of animal models were developed: *P. berghei*'s whole life cycle with *An. stephensi*; *P. cynomolgi*'s whole life cycle with *An. stephensi*; chloroquine-resistant *P. berghei* strain; and pyrimethamine-resistant *P. berghei* strain, with models for *P. berghei* and *P. gallinaceum* being developed prior to 1967. These animal models combined, could screen candidate drugs relatively accurate. In addition, China had successfully set up *in vitro* screening method for raising *An. sinensis*, *An. minimus*, *An. balabacensis*, and *An. lesteri* in laboratories.

4.2.2 Malaridine

Antimalarial drug synthesis and screening in China started before the "Mission 523". However, the "Mission 523" is credited with greatly accelerating the development of antimalarial drugs, with this area growing by leaps and bounds. From 1967 to 1981, more than 10,000 kinds of compounds were synthesized, more than 40,000 kinds of drug samples were screened, and nearly 1,000 kinds of active compounds effective for rodent malaria were found. Twenty-nine of these completed clinical verification and 14 were passed for drug appraisal (eight for new drugs and six for generic drugs).

In 1946, J. H. Burckhalter reformed chloroquine's acetaminophen side chain and synthesized amodiaquine, which showed a significant effect on malaria. In 1957, it was reported that the toxicity of 4-[(7-chloroquinolin-4-yl) amino]-2,6-bis(pyrrolidin-1-ylmethyl) phenol, named bispyroquine, was lower than that of chloroquine. In 1964, Huang Lansun and colleagues from NIPD, Shanghai, synthesized bispyroquine (code M6407).[5] In mice, its toxicity was found to be lower and its curative effect higher than that of chloroquine.[6] Inspired by this synthesis, in 1967, the Shanghai 14th Pharmaceutical Factory synthesized Pyracrine Phosphate (code 6701). It has similar characteristics to M6407. Around 1970, Zheng Xianyu used a specific side chain of M6407, and synthesized malaridine (code 7351).[7] The drug's performance was excellent, and no obvious cross-resistance with chloroquine was observed. Malaridine is highly efficient, quick acting, and has low toxicity. It is still being used to treat *P. falciparum* malaria.

4.2.3   Artemisinin

From 1967 to 1981, the "Mission 523" had many achievements, of which artemisinin is the most successful. According to statistics, various units involved in this program previously screened hundreds of medicinal herbs and obtained a batch of antimalarial activity compounds. Research journals have reported on many of these, including artemisini from *Artemisia annua* L., yingzhaosu A from *Artabotrys hexapetalus* (L.f.) Bhand, febrifugine from Dichroa febrifuga Lour, Agrimol from *Agrimonia pilosa* L., robustanol from *Eucalyptus robusta* Sm, protopine from *Nandina domestica* Thunb, bruceine D from Brucea javanica, and zincpolyanemine from Polyalthia. At first, artemisinin was not the best candidate, because other candidate drugs also had good effect when challenged against malaria infection, but taking into account both the toxicity factor and available plant resources, artemisinin finally became the best antimalarial drug during the "Mission 523" program.

Artemisia apiacea and *Artemisia annua* L are the composite plants of the *Kobresia* genus. According to literature on Chinese medicine, they have the effects of reducing fever, detoxification, and curing malaria. As early as 1600 BC, it was recorded in Li Shizhen's *Compendium of Materia Medica* that *Artemisia annua* is effective against malaria. In about 300 BC, a doctor named Ge Hong made a prescription that involved a handful of *Artemisia apiacea* in two liters water, which could treat malaria.

Tu Youyou, a researcher from the China Academy of Traditional Chinese Medicine was inspired by these Chinese traditional prescriptions. She extracted *Artemisia apiacea* with ether at a low boiling point and obtained the active ingredient, artemisinin. It was this achievement that won her the 2015 Nobel Prize in Physiology or Medicine. It is interesting to note that her name and the plant also has another connection. They appeared together in *The Book of Songs*, a well-known ancient collections of poems, from which songs were sung everywhere 2,500 years ago in China.

Due to the special structure of artemisinin, analytic work on its structure lasted for more than two years. At the end of 1975, scientists from Institute of Organic Chemistry and Institute of Biological Physics, the Chinese Academy of Sciences, finally determined the structure and absolute configuration of artemisinin, confirming that it is a sesquiterpene lactone with an endo-peroxide bridge, and this particular structure is thought to be important for its antimalarial function.[2]

Artemisinin can quickly kill parasites with minimal adverse effects, however, the relapse rates were found to be higher during emergent therapy. Artemisinin's solubility in water and oil is low, it is difficult to be storage at that time, and the oral dose is large. Due to this, researchers went on to improve two aspects. One was the dosage. Scientists developed powder, tablets, a solid dispersing agent, microcapsules, and an oil pill for oral administration. They also developed oil syringes, transparent oil suspension syringes, and water suspension syringes for injection, as well as rectal suppositories. The other aspect was to optimize the chemical structure, which involved synthesizing dihydroartemisinin, dihydroartemisinin ethers, carboxylic acid esters, carbonate and sulfonic acid esters, and more than 150 derivatives with impurity atoms. These derivatives were all found to be more effective than artemisinin to treat rodent malaria. In the end, the only derivatives chosen for clinical use were dihydroartemisinin, artemether, and artesunate, because of both the efficacy and adverse events.[3]

Artemisinin and its derivatives are efficient, quick, and have low toxicity. They have become the main drugs used to treat *P. falciparum* malaria worldwide. However, discovering artemisinin went far beyond antimalarial drug research. In China, it led to a series of research studies, from basic sciences to drug development. These included studies on pharmaceutical chemistry, plant chemistry, organic synthetic chemistry, and chemical biology. In a follow-up study, its other pharmacological effects were discovered. It demonstrated a high activity on killing the larvae of schistosomiasis in dogs and rabbits at a dose of 6 mg/kg once every 2–3 weeks.[4] Thus, artesunate and artemether were approved as schistosomiasis prevention drugs.

4.3 Schistosomicide drugs

4.3.1 Praziquantel

In 1972, praziquantel (code: Embay 8440) was synthetized by Bayer Germany. The treatment effect of praziquantel for the vast majority of parasites is quite good (85.0–100%). This resulted in Chinese research institutes synthesizing generic praziquantel in a non-for-profit manner, and conducting a lot of pharmacological research. They found that praziquantel can kill a variety of parasites in humans and animals, and especially has a significant effect on *Schistosoma japonicum*, *Clonorchis sinensis*, *Paragonimus*, *Fasciolopsis buski*, and a variety of tapeworms and their larvae. The cure rate can reach more than 90%, and it has low toxicity, a short course of treatment, and is well tolerated by patients. In addition, it is convenient for oral application, both in hospitals and in large-scale treatment at epidemic field sites. In 1984, the World Health Organization (WHO) changed the schistosomiasis control strategy from eliminating the intermediate host snails to giving priority to chemotherapy to control the source of infection. In China, the control strategy made a corresponding adjustment, in terms of expanding to repeated chemotherapy to control the source of infection.

Many researchers have studied in insecticidal mechanism of praziquantel. Xiao and colleagues have done a lot of work in this area. They thought that the parasiticidal process of praziquantel mainly includes two aspects, namely the direct effect of drugs on *Schistosoma* and the host immune effect. A small dose of praziquantel (0.01 µg/mL) can quickly cause the worm to become excited, then the worm's body becomes contracted and swollen, the cortex is roughened and seriously damaged, the function of the ventral sucker is lost, and the worm cannot stick itself in the vessel and move to the patient's liver. This movement damages the mechanism of accompany immune in the worm, exposing the epitope on the worm's body surface, then subjecting the worm to be attacked by the host's immune system, and leading to its death. The worm's body damage and its movement to the host's liver influences the worm's nutrition absorption, secretion, and defense function of the body surface and leads to metabolic disorders. It is believed that praziquantel may have a direct effect on the worm's body muscle layer and lead to the worm body's contracture.[5]

With its wide use, the issue on praziquantel resistance has begun to emerge. Praziquantel-resistant schistosomiasis strains have successfully been induced in laboratories. Therefore, in the presence of drug pressure, schistosomiasis can be resistant to praziquantel. Although praziquantel resistance to *S. japonicum* strains has not yet been found in China, *S. mansoni* was found not sensitive to praziquantel in Africa and South America, causing widespread attention. This also promotes the development of new drugs against schistosomiasis in China.[6]

4.3.2   Artemether

The treatment and control of schistosomiasis virtually relies on a single drug: praziquantel. The urgent need to develop new antischistosomal compounds has caused attention, particularly in view of widely applying of praziquantel within the framework of "preventive chemotherapy", a strategy that might select for drug-resistant parasites if praziquantel abuse used for years. Additionally, there is an important deficiency in the therapeutic profile of praziquantel. Praziquantel is not useful as a preventive drug as its actions can only last a few hours. It is effective against schistosomula for the first two days of their life, but is unable to kill them as they become mature from day 3 to day 21.

A recently developed antimalarial drug, artemether, can kill schistosomula over the period of the first 21 days following their entry into the human body. It is expected to kill all immature schistosome infections if administered every two weeks, and evidence is emerging that this is indeed the case. The drug was synthesized as β-methyl ether artemisinin by the Shanghai Institute of Materia Medica, Chinese Academy of Sciences. Although artemether first attracted people's attention for its excellent antimalarial properties, it is now known to succeed as a chemoprophylactic in the field. In a trial with residents of an endemic area, the drug was administered every 15 days throughout the transmission season at a dose of 6 mg/kg. Acute cases were prevented and infection intensity were less than half as frequent as in the control group, and were of lower intensity. Artemether is also active against other schistosome species and its overall effect is enhanced when it is combined with praziquantel. The prospects seem good for this drug to be used as a chemoprophylactic among high-risk groups, such as flood relief workers, tourists known to have been recently exposed to schistosomiasis, and fishermen, in areas of endemicity. It will probably not be deployed in areas with malaria due to fears that the low doses required for schistosomiasis prevention could enable coincident malaria organisms to develop resistance.[7]

4.4 Anti-echinococcosis drugs

4.4.1 Clinical use

Before the 1980s, surgery was the only method for the treatment of hydatid disease. However, surgery treatments might incur complications in patients who have relapsed, making surgery not suitable for all. A series of studies conducted by hard-working researchers found that benzimidazoles had a better effect on hydatid disease. Nowadays, mebendazole and albendazole are the only benzimidazole drugs used for the treatment of this disease clinically.[8]

Mebendazole was first used to treat intestinal nematodes in humans and domestic animals in 1968. In 1974, the effects of both of mebendazole and albendazole on hydatid disease were discovered. These drugs do have limitations, including poor absorption (an absorption rate of 5–10%). Mebendazole's inactive metabolites further limit its effect. Albendazole is better absorbed and its metabolite activity (sulfoxide metabolite) is also better when compared with mebendazole. Therefore, albendazole is more widely used. Since the 1980s, the WHO has conducted two multicenter clinical trials, further confirming the efficacy of the two drugs in the treatment of hydatid disease. Then from 1990s, clinical observations of mebendazole and albendazole for the treatment of hydatid disease were carried out.[9]

4.4.2　Cystic echinococcosis (CE) drugs

More than 2,000 well-documented cases of CE have been treated with benzimidazoles. When evaluated up to 12 months after initiation of chemotherapy, 10–30% of patients are cured, 50–70% are improved, and 20–30% fail treatment. Chemotherapy is suitable for inoperable patients with primary liver echinococcosis and for patients with multiple cysts in two or more organs, in which case long-term chemotherapy may be needed. Another important indication for chemotherapy is the prevention of secondary echinococcosis. The pre-surgical use of benzimidazoles may reduce the risk of CE recurring and/or facilitate the surgery by reducing intracystic pressure. However, this is not well documented.

　　Two benzimidazoles have been extensively evaluated using animal models, and the drug is recommended by the WHO.[10] The oral dosages for treatment of CE are as follows:

　　Albendazole: 10–15 mg/kg per day in two divided doses postprandially. In practice, adults should receive 800 mg/day in two single doses of 400 mg each. Clinic treatment with intervals of 14 days was originally recommended by the manufacturer, and three to six or more monthly courses have been regarded as necessary for treating patients with single or multiple cysts.

　　Mebendazole: 40–50 mg/kg per day in three divided doses for at least three to six months.

4.4.3　Alveolar echinococcosis (AE) drugs

Chemotherapy of AE in patients has been practiced since 1975. Carefully controlled clinical studies have revealed that the 10-year survival rate in inoperable or non-radically operated AE patients receiving treatment of long-term chemotherapy can be increased by 80–83% compared to 6–25% in the untreated control group.[11]

Two benzimidazoles are preferentially used for chemotherapy of AE, as described below.

Mebendazole: 500-mg tablets in daily doses of 40–50 mg/kg per day in three divided doses postprandially. After an initial continuous treatment for four weeks, it is suggested to adjust the oral doses in order to keep the plasma drug levels higher than 250 nmol/L (=74 ng/mL).

Albendazole: 400-mg tablets or 10–15 mg/kg per day in two divided doses postprandially. In practice, adults should receive 800 mg/day in two single doses of 400 mg each. Repeated cycles of 28 days' treatment should be followed by a suspension of 14 days that patients do not take albendazole.

In a review on albendazole treatment efficacy in patients worldwide with *Echinococcus granulosus*, Horton reported that the effective rate of albendazole is 75% and that of mebendazole is 58%.[12] Another report showed that albendazole and mebendazole treated 505 and 366 cases, with a cure rate of about 30%.[13]

The low solubility of benzimidazole drugs leads to poor absorption. Dawson believes that benzimidazole drug absorption difference and its characteristic of low serum concentration leads to its poor efficacy. If people can improve their bioavailability, this is expected to improve drug treatment. At present, formulations of albendazole emulsion have become commercially available, with clinical cure rates of up to 70%.[14]

4.4.4 Challenges

The major challenge in the treatment of hydatid disease is the lack of effective alternative drugs. Clinically, benzimidazole has a low cure rate and it cannot meet the need for the treatment of this disease. Research on novel compounds should be strengthened.

4.5 Drugs for other helminthiasis

Currently, first-line anthelmintic drugs are broad-spectrum, and are not only effective for treating hookworm, but also have an effect on other intestinal parasites, including soil-transmitted helminths and foodborne parasitic diseases caused by infections with *Ascaris lumbricoides*, hookworms, *Trichuris trichiura*, and pinworm.

In China, intestinal parasites are treated with generic drugs, traditional Chinese medicine, and plant extracts. Up until 1983, Chinese scientists synthesized phenylaminoamidine compounds and screened for ancylostomiasis, discovering Schiff base analogues that display good activity against *Ancylostoma* and other parasites. One of the compounds, tribendimidine, was developed into a new drug that can treat a variety of parasitic worm infestations.

4.5.1 Natural medicines and generic drugs

Before the 1970s, drugs used to treat ancylostomiasis in China mainly included chlorine hydrocarbons. There were four groups of drugs: Group 1 was carbon tetrachloride and tetrachloroethylene phenols; Group 2 was thymol 4-iodine thymol hexylresorcinol and 1-bromine-2-naphthol; Group 3 was phenylethyl ammonium salt, such as phenolic hydroxyl ethyl, ammonium naphthenate, ammonium salt, and phenylethyl gallate; and Group 4 was ether peroxide, such as ascaridole, a monoterpene containing peroxide bridge, the main component of chenopodium oil.

In 1956, a chinaberry preparation was found to have a remarkable curative effect on hookworm in the process of mass deworming of *A. lumbricoides* in primary school-aged children. During the same period, medicines used to treat intestinal nematodes in China were mainly santonin, Cortex Meliae, chenopodium oil, hexylresorcinol, tetrachloroethylene, chloroform, Oleum Ricini, and Bromine with phenol. These drugs have a narrow spectrum against intestinal nematodes, have low efficacy, and can lead to significant adverse reactions. Therefore, their use as antiparasitics was stopped one by one from the 1970s onwards.

Pagoda sugar

Pagoda sugar was a popular anthelmintic used in mass deworming of children 50 years ago. The active ingredient of the preparation was santoninum. Each piece of pagoda sugar weighed about two grams, made up of 0.04 grams of santoninum, 0.008 grams of phenolphthalein, 1.95 grams of sucrose, 0.035 grams of dry protein, 0.0001 grams of aromatic substance, 0.00005 grams of pigment, and 0.001 grams of acetate. Pagoda sugar had a conical shape and was brightly colored, and it was packaged beautifully and tasted delicious. Children loved to eat this medicine as they ordinarily love eating sweets. From the 1950s to the 1970s, pagoda sugar played a big role in protecting the health of children from parasitic infections. When the use of santoninum was stopped, researchers continuously developed other pagoda sugars with effective constituents of piperazine citrate, levamisole, or albendazole, however, these were not widely used.[15]

Generic drugs

China synthesized four generic anthelminthic drugs during the 1970s: pyrantel (1972), levamisole (1973), mebendazole (1975), and albendazole (1979). These drugs were brought into production and were used in clinical treatment after they passed drug effect and toxicity tests. Following the first national survey of important parasitic disease in China (1988–1992), many provinces (cities, districts) used the strategy of large-scale deworming with these drugs in rural areas, and especially in primary and secondary schools of these areas, coupled with health education and feces management. After nearly ten years of control, populations of *A. lumbricoides*, hookworm, and *T. trichiura* infections decreased by 71.3%, 60.7%, and 71.3%, respectively. There was a reduction to about 800 million soil-borne helminth infection cases in the 1990s in China, which shows that these strategies had made significant achievements.[16]

Albendazole

All the aforementional drugs are broad-spectrum drugs against helminths. Among them, albendazole is used most commonly in China. From 1979, albendazole had been imitated successfully. Around 28 authorized Chinese invention patents related to albendazole have been published, involving a variety of formulations and improvements of synthesis methods. In recent years, the clinical use of albendazole has taken the forms of albendazole tablets, capsules, granules, oral liquid, and dry syrup. In September 2003, an albendazole oral emulsion was launched as a fourth-grade new drug in the domestic market. It is used to clinically treat echinococcosis.

China has many albendazole manufacturers, according to incomplete statistics. In 2009, there were 39 pharmaceutical companies offering albendazole products, including the Guangzhou Pharmaceutical Factory, Shaanxi Hanjiang Pharmaceutical

Group Co., Ltd., and Tianjin Schick Pharmaceutical Group Co., Ltd. According to the *Corpus of Chinese Medicine Material* (2014 edition), 15 pharmaceutical companies have the production permit license for the active pharmaceutical ingredient of albendazole.[17]

Tribendimidine

Tribendimidine is a new drug developed in the National Institute of Parasitic Disease, China CDC, China that is a broad spectrum antihelminthic agent. It is an amidantel analogue belonging to phenylaminoamidine compounds. Amidantel was first synthesized in 1971 by Wollweber H. Animal tests showed that it was effective for many intestinal helminths such as *Ancylostoma caninum* and *Toxascaris leonina* in dogs. Amidantel has very low toxicity, and does not display any teratogenicity and mutagenicity in animal tests. When tested in clinical trials in Korea, it was shown to be effective against *Ancylostoma duodenale*, *Necator americanus*, and *A. lumbricoides* in humans.

Tribendimidine was approved by the Chinese Food and Drug Administration (CFDA) and registered as a Category I drug (a broad-spectrum antiparasitic), mostly for the treatment of hookworm disease and ascariasis on April 30, 2004. However, laboratory and clinical trials indicated that tribendimidine was effective on 21 parasites. Both animal and clinical trials showed that tribendimidine had a very significant effect on *C. sinensis* particularly.[18]

At present, to treat *C. sinensis* with praziquantel, the total recommended doses are 75–90 mg/kg, 120–150 mg/kg, and 150–180 mg/kg for light, medium, and severe infections, respectively, taken three times a day for two consecutive days. The curative effect is satisfactory, with the cure rate above 90%. However, as the dose is very large, patients comply poorly with the treatment schedule. Therefore, hospitals often reduce the dose to about 75 mg/kg. Some areas in China use albendazole to replace praziquantel. Reports show that in albendazole insecticide treatment, the total dose is 2.8 g, the period of treatment is seven days, and the cure rate is about 93.3%. Other reports show that the efficacy of 60–84 mg/kg albendazole is equal to 120 mg/kg praziquantel. Although the course of treatment with albendazole is a little longer than that of praziquantel, the adverse event rate is lower for albendazole than praziquantel. Albendazole is also highly effective against other intestinal parasites, such as *A. lumbricoides*, pinworm, and hookworm, thus this drug is fit for *C. sinensis* patients with multiple helminth infections.[19]

In rats infected with *C. sinensis*, tribendimidine was shown to have a 100% cure rate with a single dosage of 300 mg/kg, which is less than that of praziquantel (375–500 mg/kg). In a clinical trial, a good effect about 91–97% cure rate was observed in patients infected both with intestinal parasites and *C. sinensis* when treated with tribendimidine at a single dose of 400 mg. Tribendimidine is equal to a total dosage of 75 mg/kg praziquantel (three times a day for two consecutive days). It has also been reported that tribendimidine dosages of 400 mg twice a day for two days or 200 mg twice a day for three days is better than a praziquantel dosage of 600 mg three times a day for three days to treat *C. sinensis* patients.[20] As the CFDA has only authorized tribendimidine to treat hookworm disease and ascariasis, it is of utmost importance to extend its clinical application to other helminths. Shandong Xinhua Pharmaceutical Co., Ltd. is the solo manufacturer of tribendimidine.

References

1. Li RH, Rao Y, Zhang DQ. The Historical Investigation into the "523 Project" and the Discovery of Artemisinin. J of Dialectics Nature, 2013, 35(203): 108-121. (In Chinese)

2. A Detailed Chronological Record of Projuct 523 and the Discovery and Development of Qinghaosu (Artemisinin) 2nd Edition 2015, Report of 523 antimalarial research group (1967-1980): 144-149. (In Chinese)

3. Shen M, Ge HL, He YX. The immunosuppression of artemisinin. Sci Chin (B), 1983(10): 928-934. (In Chinese)

4. Li T, Chen H, Mei X, et al. The immunosuppressive and regulatory mechanism of artemisinin. Chin Pharmacol Bull, 2011, 27(6): 848-54. (In Chinese)

5. Zhou JY, Zhu Y. Progress in Antitumor Effects of Artemisinin and Its Derivatives, Nat Prod Res Dev, 2014, 26: 975-981.

6. Yang HL, Li XL, Gao BH, et al. Surveillance of *Plasmodium falciparum* susceptibility to seven antimalarials, including artemether, in the western part of the Sino-Myanmar border area. J Pathogen Biol, 2009, 4(11): 831-832

7. Liu R, Dong HF, Jiang MS. The new national integrated strategy emphasizing infection sources

control for schistosomiasis control in China has made remarkable achievements. Parasitol Res, 2013, 112(4): 1483-91.

8.　Chen YY. New integrated strategy emphasizing infection source control to curb schistosomiasis japonica in a marshland area of Hubei Province, China: findings from an eight-year longitudinal survey. PLoS One, 2014, 9(2): e89779.

9.　Xiao SH. Early treatment with artemether and praziquantel in rabbits repeatedly infected with *Schistosoma japonicum* cercariae. Zhongguo Ji Sheng Chong Xue Yu Ji Sheng Chong Bing Za Zhi, 1994, 12(4): 252-6. (In Chinese)

10.　Wu W. Clinical observation on the treatment of 1,627 cases of schistosomiasis haematobia with praziquantel of different dosages. Zhongguo Ji Sheng Chong Xue Yu Ji Sheng Chong Bing Za Zhi, 1994, 12(4): 288-90. (In Chinese)

11.　Wu W. Clinical observation on the treatment of 1,627 cases of schistosomiasis haematobia with praziquantel of different dosages. Zhongguo Ji Sheng Chong Xue Yu Ji Sheng Chong Bing Za Zhi, 1994. 12(4): 288-90.

12.　Xiao S. Effects of mebendazole, albendazole and praziquantel on alanine aminotransferase and aspartate aminotransferase of *Echinococcus granulosus* cyst wall harbored in mice. Zhongguo Ji Sheng Chong Xue Yu Ji Sheng Chong Bing Za Zhi, 1995, 13(2): 107-10. (In Chinese)

13.　Wen H. Research Achievements and Challenges for Echinococcosis Control. Zhongguo Ji Sheng Chong Xue Yu Ji Sheng Chong Bing Za Zhi, 2015, 33(6): 466-71. (In Chinese)

14.　Yu SH. Global progress of echinococcosis control and an insight to the national control program. Zhongguo Ji Sheng Chong Xue Yu Ji Sheng Chong Bing Za Zhi, 2008, 26(4): 241-4. (In Chinese)

15.　Xiao S. Effects of mebendazole, albendazole and praziquantel on alanine aminotransferase and aspartate aminotransferase of *Echinococcus granulosus* cyst wall harbored in mice. Zhongguo Ji Sheng Chong Xue Yu Ji Sheng Chong Bing Za Zhi, 1995, 13(2): 107-10. (In Chinese)

16.　Qian MB. Combating echinococcosis in China: strengthening the research and development. Infect Dis Poverty, 2017, 6(1): 161.

17.　Yan J, Hu ZL. The Endemic Situation and Challenges of Major Parasitic Diseases in China. Zhongguo Ji Sheng Chong Xue Yu Ji Sheng Chong Bing Za Zhi, 2015, 33(6): 412-7. (In Chinese)

18.　Xiao SH, Wu HM, Wang C. Tribendimidine-a new broad-spectrum drug against intestinal helminths. Zhongguo Ji Sheng Chong Xue Yu Ji Sheng Chong Bing Za Zhi, 2004, 22(5): 312-5.

19.　Xiao SH, Wu HM, Tanner M. Tribendimidine: a promising, safe and broad-spectrum anthelmintic agent from China. Acta Trop, 2005, 94(1): 1-14.

20. Zhang JH, et al. Tribendimidine enteric coated tablet in treatment of 1,292 cases with intestinal nematode infection-a phase IV clinical trial. Zhongguo Ji Sheng Chong Xue Yu Ji Sheng Chong Bing Za Zhi, 2008, 26(1): 6-9. (In Chinese)

Chapter 5

International Cooperation in Parasitic Disease Control

Ning Xiao, Jun-hu Chen, Duo-quan Wang, Ru-bo Wang, Fei Luo,

Zhi-gui Xia, Mei Li, Kun Yang, and Xiao-nong Zhou

5.1 Introduction

Globalization has had a profound impact on human health recently. In particular, transborder infectious diseases have been recognized as a global threat and an important non-traditional security issue. In respect to the fact that health is closely related to social development and justice, international communities should be obligated to eliminate health inequalities under the framework of the Millennium Development Goals (MDGs) and the post-2015 Sustainable Development Goals, proposed by United Nations. At present, two main tasks of global health are to achieve health development and maintain health security.[1]

Malaria and neglected tropical diseases (NTDs), such as schistosomiasis, are both under the heading of tropical diseases. Malaria, as the most important tropical disease in the world, exists in 109 countries and areas, and puts an estimated 3.3 billion people at risk. According to data in the 2017 World Malaria Report,[2] there were an estimated 216 million clinical malaria episodes in 2016 and an estimated 445,000 deaths. Africa is the most affected continent with nearly 90% of all malaria deaths, with Sub-Saharan Africa being particularly affected. In addition, other tropical diseases such as schistosomiasis mostly occur among neglected and marginalized communities in remote rural areas, urban slums, and conflict zones. A total of 239 million people are infected with schistosomes, with 85% of these distributed in Sub-Saharan Africa.

In recent years, as global economic growth has enhanced the status of public health, the control and prevention of NTDs has gradually received worldwide attention. In 2013, the World Health Assembly (WHA) proposed a deadline for the elimination of 10 major tropical diseases. The main challenges faced in malaria and schistosomiasis control and prevention by Asian and African developing countries are poor physical infrastructure, weak prevention and control systems, imperfect health information systems, a marked shortage of professional staff, lack of drugs/diagnostics/molluscicides/insecticides, and a huge funding gap.[3] All these insufficiencies together make it difficult to carry out effective prevention and control work in many settings.

Tropical diseases used to pose a serious burden in China. At the beginning of systematic control and prevention activities in the 1950s, the annual number of malaria cases was close to 30 million in 24 provinces, with a mortality rate of up to 1%; schistosomiasis affected an estimated 12 million people in 12 provinces. After six decades of unremitting prevention and control work, remarkable achievements have been made.

The first example is the malaria elimination program which has initiated in 2010. Malaria was an important parasitic disease that gravely influences people's health, as well as socioeconomic development. A remarkable achievement of the National Malaria Control Program (NMCP) has taken place since the early 1950s. The incidence of malaria has significantly declined from 2.4 million in the 1970s to tens of thousands by the end of the 1990s, the endemic regions have sharply shrunk, and *Plasmodium falciparum* malaria has been eliminated in all regions except for Yunnan Province in 2010. Up until 2009, the national incidence of malaria had been reduced to 14,000 in 24 malaria endemic provinces, and malaria incidence in 95% of the counties dropped below 1/10,000, with only 87 counties having a rate of over 1/10,000. The data indicate that China has transitioned from malaria control to malaria elimination.[4]

In order to respond to the global malaria elimination initiative proposed at the United Nations (UN) MDG High-level Meetings in 2010, the Chinese government launched the China action plan for the elimination of malaria in 2010, with the stated goal of eliminating indigenous malaria from most areas by 2015, except for the southern border region, and eliminating malaria nationwide by 2020.[5] The elimination strategy was defined based on epidemic levels (strata). In stratum A, where malaria incidence is above 1/10,000, control of infectious sources alongside case management and vector control should be strengthened to reduce malaria incidence. In stratum B, where malaria incidence is less than 1/10,000, infectious sources of malaria should be eliminated to block the local transmission of malaria. In stratum C, where most malaria cases are imported and sporadically distributed, surveillance and treatment of imported cases should be strengthened to prevent secondary transmission. In stratum D, considered as non-transmission areas of malaria, enhanced surveillance of imported cases is recommended. Against this strategic working plan, the number of indigenous cases has been reduced significantly down to less than 200 annually in 2015, and zero indigenous case was reported in 2017.

The second example is the National Schistosomiasis Control Program which has achieved the goal of elimination as public health problem, based or WHO criteria, by 2016. The strategy of schistosomiasis control in China since the 1980s has shifted from transmission control (targeting the snail intermediate host) to morbidity control (by means of mass chemotherapy coupled with health education), as proposed by WHO in 1984. This strategy has reduced the number of schistosomiasis patients as well as the morbidity rate remarkably since then. In the new millennium, China has shifted from mass chemotherapy to an integrated strategy with an emphasis on infection source reduction, which mainly targets fecal contamination of the environment by both humans and cattle, in the face of higher reinfection rates in transmission regions. This strategy subsided by the government for "mechanization" to replace cattle in agriculture has been very effective.[6] Until 2008, all endemic regions in China have reached the standards of disease control and were marching toward the aims of "transmission control" and "transmission interruption". Meanwhile, the control of imported schistosomiasis cases has gradually become a new focus in the country.

In summary, the malaria elimination program in China was launched in 2010, while schistosomiasis control met the goal of epidemic control nationwide in 2008, with five provinces having reached the goal of schistosomiasis elimination. Currently, malaria is expected to be eliminated by 2020, and schistosomiasis is scheduled to be eliminated by 2025, with intensively elimination program.

Health cooperation between China and other low- and middle-income countries

(LMICs) has a history of more than 50 years. At the government level, since 1963, China has dispatched 47 medical teams to Africa for medical aid, including the diagnosis and treatment of malaria and NTDs. From 2008 to 2010, China established 30 anti-malaria stations in 30 African countries to provide free antimalarial drugs and equipment, which not only played a positive role in the forming of local malaria prevention and control systems, but also fulfilled former President Hu Jintao's commitment made at the China-Africa Cooperation Forum in 2006. At the institutional level, professional institutions in China actively carry out international health cooperation in the field of research and control of malaria and schistosomiasis, which includes networking, personnel training, technical exchanges, and bilateral cooperation. Concrete activities have included taking leadership in the establishment of the Regional Network for Asian Schistosomiasis and Other Zoonotic Helminths (RNAS+) and the Chinese Network for Drugs and Diagnostics Innovation (China NDI); participating in the Asia Collaborative Training Network for Malaria (ACT Malaria); strengthening the cooperation with the regional network in Africa, such as the Regional Network for Schistosomiasis in Africa (RNSA) and the Africa NDI; and providing training courses to African scholars and professionals with a focus on infectious disease control, including control of malaria and schistosomiasis, which has benefited more than 40 African countries.[7] In addition, Chinese research institutes also offered fellowships to African researchers in China for postdoctoral training, training courses and signed memorandum of understandings (MoUs) with several LMICs (such as Sudan, Lao PDR, and Cambodia) to collaborate on research of tropical diseases. Chinese experts have been invited to Zanzibar, Uganda, Egypt, Papua New Guinea (PNG), Lao People's Democratic Republic, Cambodia, and other countries for technical consultancies and field visits to better understand local malaria and schistosomiasis situations. International symposiums and workshops on China-Africa health cooperation have been organized by leading institutions in China to discuss and explore how Chinese experiences in tropical diseases could be disseminated to LMICs in Asia and Africa.

With the expanding contributions of China's international cooperation and bilateral cooperation in the field of global health, and with the commitments for quality, applicability, and effective enhancement of China's foreign aid, a further exploration of this win-win strategy has become a pressing matter. Should this translation of Chinese experiences and lessons learned in disease control and elimination not be done in a timely manner, China (as one of the countries to witness the fastest improvements in both its economy and health status) will neither be able to take the responsibility of assisting counterpart LMICs in tackling urgent public health problems nor will it be able to make a significant contribution to global health promotion.

Initiated in 2000, MDG 6 aimed to reduce the incidence of malaria and other infectious diseases by 2015. However, lacking international aid and assistance, it is plausible to assume that the process of fighting against these public health problems will be delayed for many Sub-Saharan African countries. Correspondingly, the next step aiming at a higher standard after MDG 6 will be naturally affected in global vision.[8] Additionally, if Sub-Saharan African countries are still aiming to tackle malaria and other NTDs, and achieve the goal of control and elimination, sustainable investments from a variety of areas covering political commitment, financial support, and academic assistance are urgently required. Nonetheless, unlike financial donations, intellectual investment, including successful strategies and technologies, can empower the recipient countries to maintain the benefit even after program completion. Furthermore, already suffering from poverty and many other disadvantages, the health disparities between Sub-Saharan African regions and high-income countries will become more staggering without international support.[9] Taking malaria as an example, the gap between the incidence of selective African countries and that of China will be wider if no enhanced intervention is taken in malaria control in Africa (Figure 5.1). As such, it is of great importance that China takes the role to deliver its successful experiences to LMICs to eventually accomplish the MDG 6.[10,11]

Thus, the dissemination of synthesized and distilled Chinese experiences and technologies for tropical disease control and prevention to LMICs in Africa and Asia will not only help reduce the global disease burden, but also accelerate the elimination of malaria and schistosomiasis, and further strengthen the relevant capacity, thus helping the partner countries to achieve the SDGs agenda through a South-South cooperation approach. At the same time, through active engagement in global health, Chinese institutions will closely cooperate with high-level and multidisciplinary academic institutions in the world to strengthen international and inter-regional

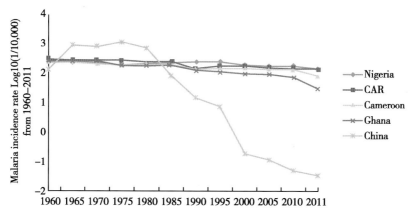

Figure 5.1   Trend in malaria log 10 incidence rate (1/10,000) in selected African countries and China, 1960–2011.

communication, dialogues, exchange, and collaboration; to enhance global health commitment and governance, as well as capacity-building; to explore global health partnerships; and to promote the health of vulnerable populations.

In this chapter, three case studies are presented along with their rationales, pre-investigation documents as well as protocols, which have trigged South-South cooperation on malaria and schistosomiasis control through multilateral cooperation. They are: (i) the China-United Kingdom (UK)-Tanzania pilot project on malaria control, (ii) the China-Australia-Papua New Guinea cooperation project on malaria control, and (iii) the China-WHO-Zanzibar cooperation project on schistosomiasis control.

5.2   Case study: China-UK-Tanzania pilot project on malaria control

5.2.1   Project title

Application of an Integrated Strategy with Community-based Approaches and Strengthening the Health System to Control Malaria Effectively in Southern Tanzania.

5.2.2   Founding and co-facilitating institutions

This project was launched in April 2015 and was completed in June 2018. It was financially supported by the Department for International Development of the United

Kingdom (UK-DFID), and co-sponsored by the Ministry of Commence of China and the National Health Commission of China. The co-facilitating institutions were the: (i) National Institute of Parasitic Diseases, Chinese Center for Disease Control and Prevention (China CDC-NIPD), Shanghai, China; (ii) Ifakara Health Institute, Tanzania; (iii) National Institute for Medical Research, Tanzania; and (iv) National Malaria Programme, Ministry of Health and Social Welfare of Tanzania.

5.2.3　Rationales

Cooperation between China and Africa in malaria control

Fifty years ago, multilateral and bilateral medical aid between China and Africa was limited. However, over the years, an amicable relationship developed between China and countries in Africa in the area of medicine and health. From 1963, when the Chinese government sent the first medical aid team to Africa, the China-Africa medical and health cooperation has grown through personal communication, the continuation of sending medical teams, conducting training of healthcare personnel, and donations of medicines and medical equipment.

Malaria cooperation between China and Africa has established mainly at the government level, and is still embodied by scientific research and academic exchanges, donations of medical equipment, and malaria control technology training. The donation of antimalarial medicines, diagnostic kits, and equipment, as well as sending experts and providing onsite training has demonstrated the Chinese government's commitment to help with malaria control and elimination in Africa. The Chinese government has helped in building anti-malaria centers in 30 African countries between 2008 and 2010. Anti-malaria centers have not only played a role in the diagnosis and treatment of malaria, but have also become centers for communication and training, which has improved the capacity of local medical research and the ability to treat the disease. Experiences with the anti-malaria centers has been faced with challenges of financing and inadequate contributions from local authorities.[12]

China also has experience in providing academic exchanges and training for African officials and technical personnel in the last 10 years. The China CDC-NIPD launched five training courses/workshops from 2013 to 2015, which were on infectious disease prevention and control, and prevention and control of malaria and schistosomiasis in Zambia, Tanzania, and Sierra Leone. More than 150 technical staff and officials from more than 20 African countries have been trained in strategy and measures of malaria prevention and control in China.

In addition, due to strong competition with well-known international pharmaceutical groups from Western countries, some of China's pharmaceutical enterprises have been successful in the process of undergoing pharmaceutical sale registration in dozens of African countries, such as Tanzania, Zambia, Kenya, and so on, providing an opportunity for the medicines to be used in the African market.

The China CDC-NIPD has also strengthened cooperation with a number of international bodies, including the Bill & Melinda Gates Foundation; the WHO; The Global Fund to Fight AIDS, Tuberculosis and Malaria; Canada's International Development Research Centre; UK-DFID; and other international agencies under multilateral or bilateral mechanisms, which is an opportunity to explore new ways of looking at malaria prevention and control. Since the Beijing Summit for China-Africa Cooperation Forum in 2006, China's support to Africa in malaria control has reached a new level.[13]

Tanzania's National Malaria Control Plan (NMCP)

National Malaria Control Plan[14]

The goal during the planning period was to reduce the average country malaria prevalence from 10% in 2012 to 5% in 2016, and to less than 1% in 2020. The following five strategic objectives support this goal:

- reduce malaria transmission by scaling up and maintaining effective and efficient vector control interventions;
- prevent the occurrence of severe morbidity and mortality related to malaria infection through the promotion of universal access to appropriate early diagnosis, prompt treatment, and provision of preventive therapies and vaccines to vulnerable groups;
- create an enabling environment in which individuals and household members are empowered to minimize their own malaria risk and seek proper and timely malaria treatment, if and when needed;
- provide timely and reliable information to assess progress in achieving

established global and national targets, to ensure that resources are used in the most cost-effective manner and to account for investments made in malaria control;

- ensure effective programmatic and financial management of malaria control interventions at all levels, implemented through effective and accountable partnerships, with adequate funding.

The plan is divided in two strategic stages: the first period (2014–2016) should sustain the recent progress and achievements; and the second period (2017–2020) will consolidate the achievements and explore the feasibility to enter into a malaria pre-elimination phase in defined areas of the country.

Achievements in national malaria control

There has been a dramatic decrease in malaria prevalence during the last strategic planning period, declining from 10% to 9.5% between 2008 and 2012. Malaria prevention through the use of insecticide-treated nets (ITNs) and long lasting insecticidal nets (LLINs) since 2009 has been successful. In addition, indoor residual spraying (IRS) has been scaled up in 18 of the 22 regions in the Lake Zone. The coverage of ITNs/LLINs has reached 14% in high transmission areas.[15]

In terms of fever management among children, there was a consistent increase in the coverage of artemisinin-based combination therapy (ACT) between 2008 and 2012, especially in rural areas. Despite the drop in malaria prevalence, the proportion of children with a history of recent febrile illness did not change. Community outreach and mobilization through radio remains the most important means of communication. However, access to messaging about malaria prevention varies greatly among groups and individuals belonging to different wealth quintiles and of different education levels.[15]

Gap analysis

Looking back, Tanzania has indeed made important progress toward ensuring access to malaria control interventions over the past years. However, there are still many challenges hindering the country reaching and sustaining a policy of universal coverage with effective curative and preventive services. Leveraging existing partnerships and effective engagement of the community in malaria control will be critical for the future of malaria control in Tanzania. Ensuring that malaria is properly diagnosed, and adequately treated and monitored will not be an easy task, however. It requires the strengthening of the health system at all levels, particularly in areas of access and quality, and especially in terms of a strong integrated surveillance system. There are reported limitations with the availability and quality of services, and even on how cases are being handled, reported, and followed up, with a lot of discrepancies between various districts.[16]

Currently, there are two primary routine reporting systems for malaria surveillance: the national Health Management Information System (HMIS) and the Integrated Disease Surveillance and Response Strategy (IDSR).[17] The HMIS is used in the health sector to collect routine data from all health facilities and it encompasses two major aspects: (i) manual routine data capturing and aggregating at the facility level (each visit to a health facility in Tanzania produces at least a single record to HMIS or IDSR health information data systems); and (ii) summary routine data entry at the district level. Malaria information collected as part of the HMIS includes rate of malaria and anemia cases among the population, and deaths in children less than five years of age and above. Most malaria cases represent clinical diagnoses that are usually non-specific fever cases. Laboratory confirmation of clinical diagnosis is conducted in all hospitals and few health centers. This information is reported annually through council health management teams and/or Health Statistics Abstract. The IDSR, on the other hand, is a strategy that assists health workers to detect and respond to diseases with epidemic potential, public health importance, and those targeted for eradication and elimination. Information from this system is intended to enable health teams to respond quickly to outbreaks, set priorities, plan interventions, and mobilize and allocate resources. In addition to the health facility- and district-based monitoring of malaria for timely action, health facility-based data collection and reporting through the electronic version of the IDSR system is also currently being implemented. However, despite the well-established presence of the two systems, which captures data from health facilities, the collected information is usually aggregated and lacks the essential breakdown by area, which is important for identifying and targeting areas of higher risk. The issue of gathering surveillance data through the IDSR system in such a way that it captures data from most health facilities including community-based approaches, needs to be strengthened through incorporating the two key parameters. Further strengthening is needed to increase the timeliness in reporting and the standardization of malaria case diagnostics.

At a time when the donor community is constrained by the global financial crisis, accessing overseas development assistance and using limited national domestic funding for malaria control will require a much stronger evidence-based business case. This is one area that the program would like to grow by learning from the Chinese experience. Based on the updated malaria control guidelines, operational manuals, and initiatives released by the WHO for scaling up diagnostic testing, treatment, and surveillance for malaria (T3),[11,18] the WHO T3 recommendation in Tanzania by adopting long-standing Chinese experiences in implementing similar strategies was evaluated. This case study report summarizes the findings of the field and desk review of the pre-evalution and designed protocol of the project in Tanzania.

International aid programs on malaria in Tanzania

(1) North-South cooperation

The following organizations and programs support Tanzania's NMCP the: United States Agency for Aid and Development (USAID), US CDCs, UK-DFID, Swiss Agency for Development and Cooperation (SDC), WHO, Swiss Tropical and Public Health Institute (Swiss TPH), Muhimbili University of Health and Allied Sciences, University of Dar es Salaam (UDSM), Johns Hopkins University COMMIT, Population Services International (PSI), Duke University of USA Mennonite Development Associates (MEDA), Clinton Health Access Initiative (CHAI), RTI International (formerly Research Triangle Institute), and John Snow Inc. (JSI).

(2) South-South cooperation

China has sent 47 medical teams to support African countries and regions in the past 50 years, providing a large number of antimalarial drugs to dozens of countries. Chinese government scholarships are established for students from developing countries to receive education in China, providing research, training, and networking opportunities for health officials, doctors, pharmacists, and scientists in Africa. As an achievement of the 2006 Beijing China-Africa Cooperation Summit, China helped build 30 hospitals in Africa with hundreds millions of dollars of artemisinin-based antimalarial drugs and to establish 30 antimalarial centers to support Africa health system.[12]

(3) International organization

The malaria program is funded by the Government of Tanzania through the Medium Term Expenditure Framework (MTEF), and is also supported by a range of partners that provide both technical and financial assistance. The main funding sources include The Global Fund, USAID/President's Malaria Initiative (PMI), WHO, and other bilateral organizations.

Although The Global Fund appears to be the main source of funding, while meetings on planning and ultimate resource allocation for the various activities/interventions outlined above are often attended by other funders to avoid overlap for a single activity. As such these different sources are integrated in some way.

China-Tanzania health cooperation

Basis for cooperation and collaboration opportunities

The China-Africa cooperation is an important part of relations between Africa and China, with the symbolic China-Africa Cooperation Forum established in 2000. Until now, the China-Africa cooperation has exhibited unprecedented depth and breadth in the field of health. In August 2013, the Ministerial Forum on China-Africa Health Development was held in Beijing, with the "Beijing Declaration of the Ministerial Forum on China-Africa Health Development" (hereinafter referred to as the "Beijing Declaration") being issued. In accordance with the Beijing Declaration, African countries decided to take a series of measures to deepen the China-Africa cooperation in health, specifically including jointly developed human resources for health and promoting the China-Africa cooperation in vocational and technical training; supporting African national health policies and programs; supporting African medicine business cooperation; encouraging technology transfer; and strengthening coordination and cooperation in global health affairs.

Importance

China has pharmaceutical, and vaccine research and development experience that may be applied in developing countries. China has accumulated some experiences and lessons in malaria prevention and control. Currently, Africa is expanding the scope and scale of health cooperation, and China is ready to share its experiences in malaria control to elimination, which can allow African countries such as Tanzania to effectively reduce the burden of malaria disease locally with local health systems.

Needs on malaria control

The future of malaria control in mainland Tanzania will depend on a carefully defined set of evidence-based objectives based on past, present, and future predictions of epidemiological conditions to target future populations for intervention packages. The proposed work will optimize the performance of the program through establishing an integrated surveillance system linking three layers of information (incidence, epidemiological, and entomological data). In addition, the project will optimize the collection, collation, and reporting of individual-level information, which is key to identifying and carefully targeting areas of higher risk. This will address the gaps highlighted in the current strategic plan, which the Tanzanian NMCP developed in 2013, in collaboration with its partners, to cover the period of 2014–2020.[14] China's experience in controlling malaria will be highly important to add value in this context.

Project significance

Combining potential resources with the local situation as well as the malaria epidemic in pilot sites of Tanzania, the China-UK-Tanzania pilot project on malaria control would explore the mode for effectively reducing local malaria disease burden by applying the WHO T3 strategy integrated with the Chinese experience in malaria control. This pilot experience will provide the impetus for developing successful customized models and experiences to control and eliminate malaria in Tanzania, while at the same time providing the platform for expanding the gained experience and successful model of aid for Africa.

5.2.4　Project design

The China-UK-Tanzania pilot program between China and Tanzania was carried out based on the successful model of the China-Africa public health cooperation, combined with local experience and technology in Africa. Its aims were to improve cooperation mechanisms between Tanzania and China, and to constantly improve the technology level and strengthen international cooperation and exchanges. The pilot needs scientific implementation of the malaria control policy, full considera- tion of local conditions, and use of various resources to reduce the local malaria burden.

Specific objectives

The specific objectives were as follows:

- To strengthen community-based interventions by adopting the WHO T3 strategy in pilot areas to: (i) increase the parasitological examination rate (T1); (ii) improve the standard treatment of confirmed and unconfirmed malaria cases (T2); and (iii) improve malaria case tracking, including case reporting and management.

- To strengthen capacity-building by establishing entomological and parasito- logical surveillance response systems, as well as information track systems, through: (i) increasing the participation of the community and partners in the control of malaria; and (ii) training local health staff and better use of exist- ing facilities.

- To strengthen the cost-effectiveness of implementing the Chinese experience in combination with the WHO T3 strategy and evaluating community-based interventions in the pilot areas, through: (i) baseline survey, mid-term assessment, and final assessment; and (ii) appraisal of pilot outputs by an external committee.

- To summarize the experiences and lessons from this collaborative pilot project and make policy recommendations for both the Chinese and Tanzanian gov- ernments.

Study areas

Rufiji was selected as the study area of this project. It is one of the six districts of the Pwani Region of Tanzania. It is bordered in the north by the Kisarawe and Mkuranga Districts, to the east by the Indian Ocean, to the south by the Lindi Region, and to the west by the Morogoro Region. The district's name comes from the Rufiji River, which runs through the district.[19]

According to the 2012 Tanzania National Census, the population of Rufiji was 217,274 (Figure 5.2). Rufiji extends from 7.470 to 8.030 south latitude and 38.620

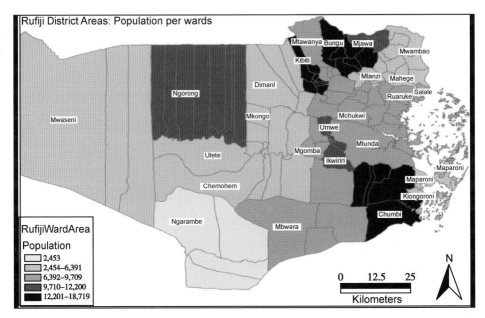

Figure 5.2   Map of Rufiji showing the population per ward (source: 2012 census data).

to 39.170 east longitude. It is located in the south of the region, approximately 178 kilometers south of Dar es Salaam, Tanzania. Rufiji has six divisions with 19 wards divided into 94 registered villages with 385 hamlets. The district covers an area of approximately 14,500 square kilometers, with an area of 1,813 square kilometers falling under the Rufiji Demographic Surveillance System that operates in six contiguous wards and 31 villages (an area of about 60 km long by 30 km wide).[20]

Rufiji has an overall mean altitude of less than 500 meters. Its vegetation is mainly tropical forests and grassland. The district has hot weather throughout the year and two rainy seasons: short rains (from October to December) and long rains (from February to May). The average annual precipitation in the district is between 800 to 1,000 millimeters. A prominent feature of the district is the Rufiji River, with its large flood plain and delta, which is the most extensive in the country. Mangrove forests flank the tributaries of the delta. The river divides the district geographically into approximately equal halves. The district is also a gateway to the Selous Game Reserve. The reserve has a variety of wild animals such as zebras, buffaloes, hartebeest, monkeys, lions, hyenas, warthogs, and elephants.[20]

The district's public health system comprises a network of more than 100 dispensaries, health centers, and hospitals, offering varying quality of care. Not all health facilities have a qualified prescriber (medical officer, assistant medical officer, clinical officer, or assistant clinical officer). Nursing cadres are responsible for preventive services such as antenatal care and well-child visits for weighing and vaccination. Some villages have volunteer village health workers.

The findings from the field visit in the pilot areas in September 2014 showed that the average malaria prevalence was more than 20% with the highest prevalence of more than 50% during the peak transmission season. The great heterogeneity of malaria prevalence arises from the ecological variation across the whole district. However, the quality of malaria diagnosis and treatment was poor due to a lack of skilled microscopists; limited supplies, including rapid diagnostic tests (RDTs) and medicine; as well as a lack of an integrated quality control and assurance system for malaria diagnosis and treatment.

References

1. Chen Z. China's Health Diplomacy. Global health 2012. Geneva, Minister of Health, People's Republic of China, 2012.

2. WHO. World Malaria Report. Global Malaria, Programme. Geneva, World Health Organization, 2018.

3. Bates I, Fenton C, Gruber J, et al. Vulnerability to malaria, tuberculosis, and HIV/AIDS infection and disease. Part 1: determinants operating at individual and household level. Lancet Infect Dis, 2004, 4: 267-277.

4. Zhou SS, Wang Y, Li Y. Malaria situation in the Peoples Republic of China in 2010, Chin J Parasitol Parasit Dis, 2011, 29(6): 401-403. (In Chinese)

5. Yin JH, Yang MN, Zhou SS, et al. Changing malaria transmission and implications in China towards National Malaria Elimination Programme between 2010 and 2012. PloS One, 2003, 8: e74228.

6. Shang LG, Wang P, Wu XW. Analyzed of the present situation and prospect of animal husbandry machinery in China, Shandong agricultural mechanization, 2013: 20-21. (In Chinese)

7. Tang LH. Progress in malaria control in China. Chin Med J, 2000, 113: 89-92. (In Chinese)

8. Cohen J, Dupas P. Free Distribution or Cost-Sharing? Evidence from a Randomized Malaria Prevention Experiment. Quart J Economi, 2010, 125(1): 1-45.

9. Marieke JW, Sandro B, Hruba F, et al. Will the European Union reach the United Nations Millennium declaration target of a 50% reduction of tuberculosis mortality between 1990 and 2015? BMC Public Health, 2017, 17: 629.

10. WHO. World Malaria Report. Global Malaria, Programme. Geneva, World Health Organization, 2010.

11. WHO. World Malaria Report. Global Malaria, Programme. Geneva, World Health Organization, 2012.

12. Shuang L, Liang MG, Reyes M, et al. China's health assistance to Africa: opportunism or altruism? Globalization and Health, 2016, 12: 83.

13. Pei LL, Yan Guo. et al. China's distinctive engagement in global health. Lancet, 2014. 384: 793-804.

14. Ministry of Health and Social Welfare-Tanzania. Tanzania National Malaria Strategic Plan, 2013, 2014-2020.

15. NMCP. National Malaria Control Programme (NMCP, Ministry of Health & Social Welfare (MoHSW) (2012). Malaria Programme Performance Review Tanzania Mainland. MoHSW, United Republic of Tanzania, April 2012.

16. NBS. Tanzania HIV and Malaria Indicator survey 2011/12 Dar es Salaam, GoT.

17. US. President's Malaria Initiative. Tananazia Malaria Operational Plan FY, 2017.

18. WHO. World malaria report 2013. Geneva, World Health Organization, 2013.

19. Kabula B, Tungu P, et al. Susceptibility status of malaria vectors to insecticides commonly used for malaria control in Tanzania. Trop Med Int Health, 2012, 17: 742-750.

20. MRA&LG. Ministry of Regional Administration & Local Government (MRA&LG). Policy paper on Local Government reform. Ministry of Regional Administration & Local Government, United Republic of Tanzania, October 1998.

5.3 Case study: Australia-China-Papua New Guinea (PNG) malaria project

5.3.1 Project title

Australia-China-PNG Pilot Cooperation on Malaria Control in Papua New Guihea (PNG).

5.3.2　Founding and co-facilitating institutions

The Funding for the project was provided by both the Australian and Chinese governments, and co-facilitated by various institutions. These institutions include National Department of Health (NDoH), PNG; the PNG Institute of Medical Research (IMR); Central Public Health Laboratory (CPHL), PNG; School of Medical and Health Sciences (SMHS), University of PNG; Health and Human Immunodeficiency Virus (HIV) Implementation Services Provider (HHISP), Australia; National Health Comnission (NHC), China; Ministry of Commence (MoFCOM), China; National Institute of Parasitic Diseases at Chinese Center for Disease Control and Prevention (China CDC-NIPD), China; Yunnan Institute of Parasitic Diseases, China; Shangdong Institute of Parasitic Diseases, China; Chongqing Certer for Diesease Control and Prevention, China; and Australian Army Malaria Institute (AMI), Australia.

5.3.3　Rationales

Accurate diagnosis of malaria is critical for determining the appropriate course of treatment and for providing accurate data to the National Health Information System (NHIS). In PNG, malaria is diagnosed using rapid diagnostic tests (RDTs) and/or light microscopy. Between 2004 and 2014, an intensified malaria control program has significantly increased the coverage of long lasting insecticidal nets (LLINs) in the country,[1] as well as the coverage of artemisinin-based combination therapies (ACTs).[2] These interventions, especially the distribution of LLIN, have led to a significant overall reduction in the prevalence (2009: 12%; 2014: 2% by light microscopy) and clinical incidence (2009: 20.5%; 2014: 4.8% at four sentinel sites) of malaria nationwide.[3] However, subnational data illustrated distinct response dynamics in different parts of the country (Figure 5.3) despite the standardized approach to rolling out malaria control interventions. A swift reduction was observed in traditionally marginal areas of the highlands fringe (Karimui), whilst in Madang province the downward trend has slowed down since 2013 and may have even reversed.

　　Despite these impressive reductions, the challenges for sustained malaria control and progress towards malaria elimination in PNG remain substantial.[3] The key challenge amongst them is the highly heterogeneous nature of malaria as transmis-

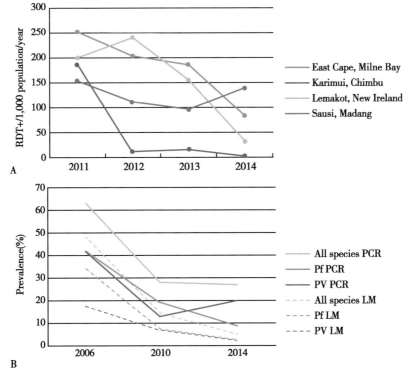

Figure 5.3   (A) Malaria incidence in sentinel health facilities and (B) malaria prevalence in project study sites on the north coast of Madang. Dots indicate year of LLIN distribution.

sion declines, which requires targeted control measures in addition to sustaining current levels of coverage with preventative and curative interventions. With regards to case management, challenges include point-of-care screening for glucose-6-phosphate dehydrogenase (G6PD) status for effective treatment of *Plasmodium vivax* with primaquine, health worker adherence to diagnostic algorithms and treatment protocols, as well as asymptomatic and submicroscopic infections, which are generally undetected by existing surveillance/control programs and now account for the overwhelming majority of infections in areas of low endemicity, thus contributing to ongoing residual transmission.[4]

The components included in the project's operational research protocol are focused on addressing some of the key challenges related to malaria case management, particularly diagnostic aspects. The project has not only provided much needed evidence for the PNG's National Malaria Control Program (NMCP), regarding effective integration of possible solutions into it, but has also led to skills transfer and capacity-building for the CPHL, PNG IMR, NDoH, and other relevant (national and subnational) stakeholders. In particular, a clear aim was defined within this program to ensure opportunities for medical registrars, and public health students and personnel to gain experience in conducting operational research. It is noted that China CDC-NIPD has significant expertise and resources to be shared in key areas outlined in the project's research protocol and the project has drawn upon the China CDC-NIPD's comparative advantage as appropriate during implementation.

5.3.4　Project design

Objective

The project aimed for a collaborative operational research of practical value to improve the quality of malaria diagnosis and, ultimately, overall case management and surveillance in PNG.

Study areas

The PNG IMR has established malaria sentinel surveillance sites for the monitoring of trends in malaria indicators since 2010.[5] The operational research design has utilized four of these sites (Lemakot, Sausi, Karimui, and East Cape) as the platform upon which to address some or all the priority research questions. This design aimed to utilize the advantages of existing collaborative set-ups and local capacity, and allow for rapid start-up within the existing sites. Furthermore, the sites may provide high quality longitudinal background data from all the four regions, which is essential to contextualizing findings of the operational research. In order to reduce operational and financial resource implications, a sampling approach was adopted for some questions, whilst ensuring the effectiveness of the study.

5.3.5　Primary research activities

Health facility surveillance of febrile illness

As transmission declines, routine surveillance must be able to adequately identify foci of residual transmission. Ongoing surveillance points to substantial heterogeneity at the local level, but it remains unclear how well RDTs or microscopy-based diagnosis can predict areas with residual parasitemia as detected by polymerase chain reaction (PCR), and whether there are differences in this ability between geographical areas and parasite species. As PNG's control program matures to an elimination stage, this information is required to interpret NHIS data and develop its surveillance approach for targeting interventions.

Study aims:

- To describe trends in malaria incidence by parasite species and understand the relative diagnostic performance of RDTs, microscopy, and PCR in the detection of malaria infection in the study sites.
- To validate the testing of pregnant women during antenatal care visits to predict population prevalence of malaria.

Comparison of the WHO-approved malaria RDTs (mRDTs)

Given the high reliance on mRDTs for diagnosis of malaria in PNG and the lack of access to high-quality microscopy in the majority of health facilities across the country, it is important for the NMSP to confirm the performance and suitability of the current mRDT. The mRDT that is currently in widespread use across PNG is the *CareStart*™ Malaria HRP2/pLDH (Pf/PAN) Combo, which detects histidine-rich protein 2, HRP2 (expressed only by *P. falciparum*) and plasmodium lactate dehydrogenase, pLDH (expressed by *P. falciparum*, *P. vivax*, *P. ovale*, and *P. malariae*). It is therefore capable of detecting the presence of all four *Plasmodium* species endemic in PNG.

This diagnostic is the WHO-approved mRDT that scores well for the detection of both *P. falciparum* and *P. vivax* infections.[8] However, this test cannot differentiate between mixed infections of *P. falciparum* and non-*P. falciparum* species, and pure *P. falciparum* infections. Many infections are therefore being diagnosed as mixed *P. falciparum*/*P. vivax* infections that are likely not mixed infections. In particular, the increasing burden of *P. vivax* requires considering potential alternatives to Pan RDTs (the RDT that detects all the four types of plasmodia that infect humans). In addition, newer tests have come onto the market in the period since the implementation of this test and so it is timely to confirm whether this mRDT is still the most appropriate one for PNG.

Study aims:

- Elaboration of consensus document on the ideal characteristics of mRDTs for implementation in the PNG context.

- Comparative assessment of two to three mRDTs for ability to (a) differentiate mixed *P. falciparum* and non-*P. falciparum* species infection from pure *P. falciparum* infections, and (b) diagnose low-density *P. vivax* infections.

- Qualitative study on health workers acceptability/ease of use and interpretation of the two to three mRDTs.

Molecular diagnosis

Routine diagnosis of malaria at health-facility level is based on RDTs. While these tests have been shown to have sufficient sensitivity to detect clinical cases requiring or those not requiring immediate antimalarial treatment,[9] they are unable to detect very low level (and potentially not disease causing) parasitemia, which contributes to ongoing transmission. At the same time, the sensitivity of RDTs currently in use in PNG might be compromised if parasites lacking the HRP2 gene are present.[10] Parasite genetic diversity studies are a powerful tool to guide malaria control and elimination strategies by tracing routes of transmission and the sources of epidemics,[11-13] and by identifying defined geographic clusters with limited gene flow, as such, the risk of reintroduction may be the lowest.[11, 14] Assuming imported cases are also antigenically distinct from local cases, imported infections may be more likely to be found in symptomatic cases than asymptomatic cases. In addition to developing malaria PCR capacity at the CPHL as part of this research component, there is also an urgency to establish routine population-level PCR malaria screening at the CPHL/NDoH.

Study aims:

- Compare RDT, microscopy, and quantitative PCR results on a subset of clinical samples in order to understand the relative sensitivity of routinely applied RDT (and microscopy).

- Investigate samples from RDT-negative/PCR-positive individuals for the presence of parasites with HRP2 deletions.

- Investigate population genetics in selected samples to establish the origin of cases in hotspots: whether they are imported or local transmission.

Point-of-care G6PD screening/testing

Glucose-6-phosphate dehydrogenase deficiency is a heritable condition that can cause hemolytic anemia in individuals, leading to hemolysis when exposed to various oxidative stresses including antimalarial drugs such as primaquine.[18] Primaquine is especially important in the treatment and control of *P. vivax* malaria. Identifying individuals with a G6PD deficiency allows for tailored treatment regimens of primaquine that are likely to be safer than the standard prescribed course.[18] Effective use of primaquine is an integral part of the national policy for malaria control, elimination, and prevention. Identifying individuals with a G6PD deficiency directly impacts on the use of primaquine treatment for *P. vivax* malaria for that individual. This information may allow treating clinicians to customize primaquine doses for each patient, thus greatly increasing the safety of this treatment.

Study aims:

- To establish local capacity for point-of-care G6PD diagnostic testing at the sentinel sites and for high quality quantitative G6PD testing at the CPHL.
- To determine the feasibility of using newly developed point-of-care G6PD diagnostic tests at the health center-level compared to quantitative testing performed at the CPHL.
- To generate G6PD prevalence data from the study sites to add to the national and regional prevalence data of severe and intermediate G6PD deficiency in PNG.
- To assess health worker perceptions on point-of-care G6PD testing and primaquine treatment.

Behavior of health workers

Compliance to febrile case management protocols can be improved through the development of health worker informed interventions. Health worker compliance with the PNG National Malaria Treatment Protocol has been monitored by repeat, countrywide cross-sectional surveys since 2010. Findings from these surveys indicate that a substantial change in malaria case management has taken place since the introduction of the test-and-treat malaria protocol. The use of mRDTs to test for malaria infection in febrile patients increased from 16.2% in 2010 to 68.3% in 2012, whereas antimalarial prescriptions given to this patient group decreased from 96.4% in 2010 to 38.0% in 2012.[2, 19] However, health worker compliance remains problematic in some areas. For example, not all febrile patients are tested for malaria infection by mRDT or microscopy; obsolete antimalarials continue to be prescribed to presumptively or clinically diagnosed malaria cases or patients testing negative for malaria infection by mRDT, and primaquine is often not prescribed to patients with a non-*P. falciparum* malaria infection or a mixed *P. falciparum* infection.[20] In addition, an analysis of health worker practices conducted in the 12-month period immediately following the introduction of the test-and-treat protocol strongly suggests health workers are often incorrectly diagnosing and treating non-malaria febrile illnesses (NMFIs) when a malaria infection has been ruled out by mRDT.[21]

Study aims: Poor health worker adherence/compliance to diagnostic and treatment protocols may be associated with a lack of motivation due to a lack of education, training, and supervisory visits. This component might therefore entail a detailed analysis and dissemination of the available quantitative data pertaining to health worker compliance with recommended febrile case management protocols. This may inform and be utilized in a pilot activity conducted by the NDoH and CPHL in selected locations in the country to raise awareness, conduct refresher training sessions, and encourage behavior change and adherence to diagnostic and treatment protocols.

Investigating use of foci to identify asymptomatic reservoirs of infection

Asymptomatic and submicroscopic infections, which are undetected in existing surveillance/control programs, now account for the overwhelming majority of infections in areas of low endemicity.[4] Understanding the prevalence and spatial distribution of asymptomatic malaria infections, particularly in relation to clinical cases and foci, and developing the capacity to identify such hotspots might be essential for the NMCP's ability to progress towards more targeted interventions in the future.

Study aims: To identify asymptomatic reservoirs of malaria infections to improve the ability of the NMCP to conduct intervention properly.

Investigating NMFI

Following the rollout of mRDTs and associated training for health workers, diagnostic training has not received sufficient resourcing in recent years to enable follow-up training in identified problem areas. Given that high levels of clinical diagnosis of malaria/presumptive treatment still remain, assisting health workers in improving diagnosis of non-malaria febrile episodes contributes to improving overall malaria diagnosis and treatment. However, this is a highly complex and extensive area requiring the collection of very detailed clinical data to accompany any additional laboratory testing for underlying causes of NMFIs. Investigated diseases would need to be prioritized given the long list of non-malaria febrile causes, and varying seasonal and geographic factors.

Study aims: To strengthen skilled experiences and confidence in diagnosing and treating NMFIs by linking into the development of revised diagnostic training aides/ manuals and future health worker training programs.

5.3.6　Evaluation

Laboratory evaluation

Diagnosis of malaria by light microscopy

Thick and thin smears are required to be prepared by research assistants at the sentinel sites. The presence of *Plasmodium* spp. is determined by light microscopy using standard PNG IMR protocols, i.e. independent read of all slides by two microscopists, with a third read to resolve any discrepancies. Evaluation of the blood smear is performed by examining a total number of oil immersion fields to include 200/500 leukocytes depending on the density of infection, with the assumption that the mean leukocyte count is 8,000 per microliter of blood. Results are expressed as the number of asexual parasites per microliter of blood.

DNA extraction for PCR analysis

In order to obtain high-quality DNA for genomic analysis, DNA from blood samples are extracted using protocols established at PNG IMR in Madang. The utility of the DNA is to confirm and characterize the *Plasmodium* spp. infection and investigate the presence of deletions in *P. falciparum* HRP2.

Diagnosis of malaria by PCR

As each individual's genomic DNA preparation contains both human and parasite DNA, blood samples can be used to perform species-specific quantitative real-time PCR diagnosis of *Plasmodium* spp. infection, which is established at the PNG IMR, however, this is planned to be developed at the CPHL during the course of this project.

Collaboration and capacity development

Technical leaders have agreed that the research protocol should maximize collaboration with existing national stakeholders (e.g. the CPHL, NDoH, SMHS), and research and development partners (Burnet Institute and the WHO). Technical leads noted the importance of using this research to provide training and capacity-building of PNG IMR, CPHL, NDoH, SMHS, and other stakeholders, to maximize opportunities to build the skills of PNG staff. Phase 1 of the study (two months) involves a comprehensive consultation with all stakeholders—the NDoH, SMHS, CPHL, NIPD, PNG IMR, NMCP Technical Working Group (TWG), WHO, AMI— to discuss the priorities of this capacity development and to make arrangements for the involvement of medical registrars, public health students, and the NDoH MSCU. Based on the outcomes of this design work, PNG IMR will work with the technical leaders to develop a work plan that identifies the specific areas and methods for the involvement of these personnel.

5.3.7   Quality assurance

This study is conducted according to the procedures outlined in the project. In order to assure both compliance with the project's protocol and assure the quality of the data collected, local quality control procedures are put in place. The different tasks to be performed in the field and laboratory are defined in specific standard operating procedures (SOPs). Adherence to both the project's protocol and SOPs is monitored via regular spot checks on collection of primary field data, checks of all forms by study coordinator or designee upon receipt from field teams, double reading of all blood slides collected, and regular data audits following second entry into all databases. In addition, senior investigators are required to regularly perform internal audits that assess completeness and accuracy of study files, CRFs, and source documents, as well as the ethical standards of study operations.

All specimens collected, as well as their transfer between different sites, are recorded in a specimen logbook. The site laboratory investigators are required to regularly check lab books and documents to assure compliance with laboratory SOPs. The detailed quality control and quality assurance procedures will be set out in specific SOPs for quality management.

5.3.8   Informed consent

During routine morbidity surveillance in sentinel site health facilities, individual informed consent will be sought for procedures that go beyond the routine work of the participating health facilities. On occasions in which finger-prick blood samples or buccal samples are collected, the participants are asked to confirm their consent by signing or writing their initials in a provisioned space on the data collection sheet. For children under 16 years of age, consent are obtained from a parent or guardian.

For participation in any household surveys, individual written informed consent is sought from all participants prior to the collection of any data. For children under 16 years of age, written informed consent is obtained from a parent or guardian.

Participation in all studies is completely voluntary and refusal to participate does not result in any negative consequences. Particularly, the participation of a village or an individual will not have any influence on the implementation of any malaria control interventions, e.g. the distribution of mosquito nets.

Prior to conducting a household survey, community meetings (*toksaves*) are held in all participating villages. These meetings serve to communicate the purpose of the study and answer questions at the individual and community level. In particular, villagers were informed about the confidentiality of the data collected and about the purpose of taking finger-prick blood samples. Samples are only used for the purpose communicated to the participants. Permission to conduct the survey in a particular location was sought from the respective village leaders.

5.3.9   Data management

Data collection forms and management
Data collection forms
Simple data collection forms developed in Round 3 Malaria Control Program Evaluation Plan for continuous morbidity monitoring at sentinel site health facilities continue to be used for routine morbidity surveillance.

Data management

All paper forms are sent to PNG IMR in Goroka where data are double entered by trained data entry clerks into the REDCap software. The master database is housed on the server in Goroka and backed up monthly to disks or other media. All paper forms are stored in lockable filing cabinets as described under.

Data analysis

Data analyses are performed using Stata (StataCorp LP, College Station, TX, USA) or SAS (Cary, NC, USA). Univariate analysis are performed to describe demographic and baseline characteristics of the study samples. The distribution of impact and outcome variables are compared across demographic characteristics (province, age, sex, SES), reported and measured intervention coverage, and across individuals in communities before, during, and after the implementation of different interventions. Bivariate analyses include chi-square tests to assess dichotomous variables, Mann-Whitney U tests to compare non-normally distributed continuous data, and *t*-tests to compare normally distributed continuous data. Statistical analyses are used to estimate the magnitude of the effect of the implemented interventions on impact indicators. Hypothesis testing are used to determine whether or not absolute and relative target values of outcomes and impact indicators have been achieved. Multivariate logistic models are used to control for covariates and to estimate the relative effect of several factors on outcome and impact measurements.

Data dissemination and reporting

Technical leads are required to ensure close liaison with the PMG Malaria TWG through participation in fortnightly TWG meetings and using these meetings to provide continuous updates on research progress and initial findings. Six-monthly reports will be submitted to the PNG Malaria TWG, the Trilateral Malaria Project (via the project manager), and other relevant stakeholders. Data will be presented in text, tabular, and graphic formats. Statistical analyses will include univariate summaries, test statistics, magnitude of effect estimates, standard error/confidence intervals, and measures of statistical significance, as appropriate.

Quarterly meetings of technical leads are planned to held in line with six-monthly Joint Project Working Group meetings, and include a review of research progress and initial findings, as well as a discussion of operational research needs.

In addition, results generated from this project will be published in a timely manner in peer-reviewed scientific journals and will be used in presentations at national and international scientific meetings. No findings will be presented or published without the agreement of all principal and co-investigators named in this project. In particular, the investigators will actively seek to involve PNG staff and students as co-authors in all publications, and as lead authors when possible. Authorship guidelines will be as inclusive as possible, with individuals who are actively involved in implementing the research project and analyzing the data named and all investigators of this project named in every presentation and publication under the banner of "Australia-China-PNG Pilot Cooperation on Malaria Control Project".

Opportunities for public dissemination of key findings for the information of the interested general public (such as through domestic and international media outlets) will be pursued where possible. The investigators (and co-authors) will seek approval from all relevant stakeholders prior to any media activity or release.

References

1. Hetzel M, Pulford J, Gouda H, et al. The Papua New Guinea National Malaria Control Program: Primary Outcome and Impact Indicators, 2009–2014. Goroka: Papua New Guinea Institute of Medical Research, 2014.

2. Pulford J, Kurumop SF, Ura Y, et al. Malaria case management in Papua New Guinea following the introduction of a revised treatment protocol. Malar J, 2013; 12: 433.

3. Cotter C, Sturrock H, Hsiang M, et al. The changing epidemiology of malaria elimination: new strategies for new challenges. Lancet, 2013; 382: 900-11.

4. Bousema T, Okell L, Felger I, et al. Asymptomatic malaria infections: detectability, transmissibility and public health relevance. Nat Rev Microbiol, 2014; 12: 833-840.

5. Hetzel M, Maraga S, Reimer L, Barnadas C, et al. Evaluation of the Global Fund-supported National Malaria Control Program of Papua New Guinea 2009–2014. PNG Med J, 2014; 57: 7-29.

6. van Eijk AM, Hill J, Noor AM, et al. Prevalence of malaria infection in pregnant women compared with children for tracking malaria transmission in sub-Saharan Africa: a systematic

review and meta-analysis. Lancet Glob Heal, 2015; 3: e617-28.

7. Kelly G, Hale E, Donald W, et al. A high-resolution geospatial surveillance-response system for malaria elimination in Solomon Islands and Vanuatu. Malar J, 2013; 12.

8. WHO. Recommended selection criteria for procurement of malaria rapid diagnostic tests. Glob Malar Program, 2016.

9. Senn N, Rarau P, Manong D, et al. Rapid diagnostic test-based management of malaria: an effectiveness study in Papua New Guinean infants with *Plasmodium falciparum* and *Plasmodium vivax* malaria. Clin Infect Dis, 2012; 54: 644-651.

10. Cheng Q, Gatton ML, Barnwell J, et al. *Plasmodium falciparum* parasites lacking histidine-rich protein 2 and 3: a review and recommendations for accurate reporting. Malar J, 2014; 13.

11. Bousema T, Griffin JT, Sauerwein RW, et al. Hitting hotspots: spatial targeting of malaria for control and elimination. PLoS Med, 2012; 9: 1-7.

12. Takala S, Plowe C. Genetic diversity and malaria vaccine design, testing and efficacy: preventing and overcoming "vaccine resistant malaria". Parasite Immunol, 2009; 31: 560-573.

13. Ghansah A, Amenga-Etego L, Amambua-Ngwa A, et al. Monitoring parasite diversity for malaria elimination in sub-Saharan Africa. Science, 2014; 345: 1297-1298.

14. Schultz L, Wapling J, Mueller I, Ntsuke PO, et al. Multilocus haplotypes reveal variable levels of diversity and population structure of *Plasmodium falciparum* in Papua New Guinea, a region of intense perennial transmission. Malar J, 2010; 9: 336.

15. Wampfler R, Mwingira F, Javati S, et al. Strategies for detection of *Plasmodium* species gametocytes. PLoS One, 2013; 8: e76316.

16. Rosanas-Urgell A, Mueller D, Betuela I, et al. Comparison of diagnostic methods for the detection and quantification of the four sympatric *Plasmodium* species in field samples from Papua New Guinea. Malar J, 2010; 9: 361.

17. Hofmann N, Mwingira F, Shekalaghe S, et al. Ultra-sensitive detection of *Plasmodium falciparum* by amplification of multi-Copy subtelomeric targets. PLoS Med, 2015; 12: 1-21.

18. Carson P, Flanagan C, Ickes C, et al. Enzymatic deficiency in primaquine-sensitive erythrocytes. Science, 1956; 124: 484-5.

19. Pulford J, Mueller I, Siba PM, et al. Malaria case management in Papua New Guinea prior to the introduction of a revised treatment protocol. Malar J, 2012; 11: 157.

20. Pulford J, Smith I, Mueller I, et al. Health worker compliance with a "test and treat" malaria case management protocol in Papua New Guinea. PLoS One, 2016; 11: e0158780

21. Saweri O, Pulford J, Mueller I, et al. The treatment of non-malaria febrile illness in Papua New Guinea: findings from cross sectional and longitudinal studies of health worker practice. BMC Heal Serv Res,2017; 17: 10.

5.4 Case study: China-WHO-Zanzibar schistosomiasis project

5.4.1 Project title

The China Aid Project of Schistosomiasis Control and Elimination in Zanzibar

5.4.2 Founding and co-facilitating institutions

This project was financially supported by the Ministry of Commence (MoFCOM) of China, co-facilitated by the Jiangsu Institute of Parasitic Diseases, the Ministry of Health of Zanzibar, and the WHO's Department of Control of Neglected Tropical Diseases.

5.4.3 Rationales

Schistosomiasis is a global public health problem, and there are 78 endemic countries and regions in Asia, South America, the Middle East, and Africa. The 2009 WHO report showed that there were 800 million people at risk of schistosomiasis, and nearly 239 million people were infected with schistosomiasis, 85% of who were in Sub-Saharan Africa. The death estimates due to schistosomiasis varied between 10,100, and 200,000 globally per year. This should has decreased considerably due to the impact of scaling up large-scale preventive chemotherapy campaigns over the past decade. Estimates show that at least 206.5 million people required preventive treatment for schistosomiasis in 2016, out of which more than 88 million people were reported to have been treated. [1,2]

Schistosomiasis was one of the most serious parasitic diseases in China, with a documented history of over 2,100 years. During the mid-1950s, at the beginning of the national control program, schistosomiasis was endemic in 12 provinces, with an estimated 11.6 million people and 1.2 million cattle infected, and an area of

14,300 km^2 infested by the intermediate host snail. Up until now, China has been successful in the control and elimination of schistosomiasis. According to the actual situation and the medium- and long-term planning goals from 2004 to 2015, a new integrated strategy to mainly target the source of transmission, such as water baffalo, was implemented in China.[3, 4] Many pilot control strategies focused on intermediate host snails, as well as on diagnosis and treatment of cases have been successfully achieved, thus providing strong knowledge and technology support for achieving the goal of the national control program. All endemic counties reached the criteria of infection control by the end of 2010, and achived the criteria of transmission control by 2016.[5-9] At the same time, China trained many experts and accumulated rich experience on the comprehensive control of schistosomiasis transmission.[10]

In 2012, the World Health Assembly (WHA) adopted a resolution on the elimination of schistosomiasis (WHA65.21).[11] The WHO has started the process of finalizing a revised global strategy as roadmap for schistosomiasis elimination including control of morbidity, elimination as a public health problem, and interruption of schistosomiasis transmission.[12] In 2014, the WHO signed a tripartite Memorandum of Understanding (MoU) with China and Zanzibar, paving the way for a pilot schistosomiasis elimination program in Zanzibar. The pilot study has been implemented on Pemba Island for three years. The goal of the study was to understand the transmission pattern of schistosomiasis, and formulate control strategies and measures based on local conditions integrated with China's experience of schistosomiasis control.

5.4.4　Project design

Objectives

The aim of the project is to promote the control and elimination program on schistosomiasis in Pemba Island, Zanzibar, with the following specific aims:

- To understand the transmission pattern of schistosomiasis in Pemba Island based on studies both in laboratory and field.
- To build and improve the capacity of schistosomiasis control via training of Zanzibar's staff and provision of equipment.
- To design control strategies and measures based on local conditions as well as experiences from China, and then implement them in a pilot region.

- To explore cooperation mechanisms between China, Africa, and the WHO in order to control and eliminate schistosomiasis in Africa.

Study area

Zanzibar, composed of two sister islands (Unguja and Pemba), is situated off the eastern cost of Tanzania's mainland. The northern tip of Unguja Island is located at 5.72 degrees south, 39.30 degrees east, with the southernmost point at 6.48 degrees south, 39.51 degrees east. The northern tip of Pemba Island is located at 4.87 degrees south, 39.68 degrees east, and the southernmost point is located at 5.47 degrees south, 39.72 degrees east.[13] Zanzibar consists of five administrative regions: three in Unguja and two in Pemba. Each region is composed of two districts, which means there are 10 districts in Zanzibar.

The island of Pemba was selected as a pilot study region. It is divided into two regions (south and north) and four districts (Figure 5.4). Each district is divided into small administrative *shehias*, with a total of 132. The western half of the island and

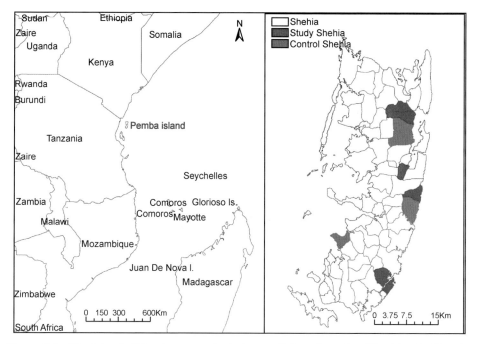

Figure 5.4   The island of Pemba was selected as a pilot study region. The island of Pemba is divided into two regions (south and north) and four districts.

the south tip are broken up into many valleys, all densely covered with clove and coconut plantations interspersed with food and crops. The largest permanent pond is found in the central-east parts of the island, while there are small ones are in the northwest. The climate is characterized by dry and rainy seasons, with the rainy seasons usually from mid-March to mid-June and from November to December. Average annual temperatures range from 23°C to 28°C.

The estimated total resident population in Unguja and Pemba was 773,234 and 500,600 inhabitants, respectively, in 2010. Islam is the predominant religion. The main economic activities include seawater fishing and cash crop production. The average number of school-aged children per study household was 1.9, without significant differences observed between *shehias* (range 1.8–2.3). A wide variation in the proportion of non-enrolled students (19–84%) was observed between *shehias*.[14]

Zanzibar is endemic for *Schistosoma haematobium*. The distribution of schistosomiasis in Unguja and Pemba was first described in 1925 (Aders, 1928). Two types of snails were responsible for transmission, namely *Bulinus nasutus*, which prefers swamps and slow flowing rivers that retain residual water for most of the year, and *B. globosus*, which prefers streams and permanent water bodies. The latter seem to be more widely distributed than the former on the Pemba Island. *Bulinus forskalii* seems to be refractory to infection in comparison with the local streams of *S. haematobium*.[15, 16] In 1975, it was estimated that 60% of the Pemba population either had intestinal schistosomiasis or had urinary schistosomiasis and that about 10% of those infected had associated morbidity. In 1981, data revealed that the infection rates of school-aged children were 65% and 70% in Unguja and Pemba, respectively. By 2004, the infection rates of schistosomiasis reduced to 49.8% and 64.5%.[17–19] In 2011, a survey of 24 schools showed that the infection rates dropped to 8% (0–38%) and 15% (1–43%) in Unguja and Pemba, respectively.[16]

5.4.5   Research activities

This study is conducted for three years, with the timeline shown in Figure 5.5. During the course of implementation, an annual evaluation is conducted to track the progress of the study and determine if any adjustments to the interventions are needed.

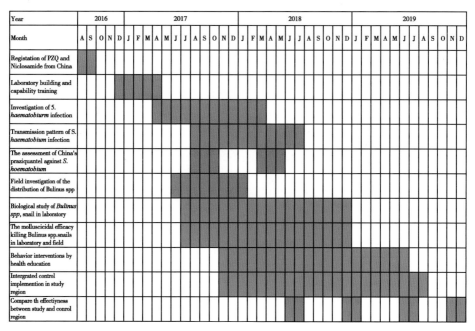

Figure 5.5   The timeline of China-WHO-Zanzibar schistosomiasis project.

Historical data collection and questionnaire survey

Historical data from the last five years have been collected, including: demographic, economic, and hydrographic characteristics; distribution of *Bulinus* spp. snail populations; number of human infections with *S. haematobium*; and the implementation of control interventions. Fifty households randomly selected from each pilot site participated in the questionnaire survey, with household- and individual-level information collected. Household-level information included family composition, economic status, type of water used, and children's school enrollment. Individual-level information included age, sex, occupation, production and lifestyle, lavatory facilities and presence of *S. haematobium* infection and treatment. In addition, the households location are recorded by using the global positioning system (GPS).

Field investigation of the distribution of *Bulinus* spp. snails

All aquatic snails were captured in suspected *Bulinus* spp. habitats each month of the first year, and the number of *Bulinus* spp. snails was counted after morphological identification. The distribution and density of *Bulinus* spp. snails were investigated, with the infection detected by microscopy. The suspected habitats are positioned using GPS. The hydrographic and environmental characteristics of the investigated areas were collected during the snail survey with the length, width, and water flow velocity of the river and pond measured. In addition, fluctuations of water areas were investigated. A database on hydrological and snail status were established, and the distribution of *Bulinus* spp. snails is mapped using Google Earth. The snail distribution area and range are investigated in both dry and rainy seasons, with the distribution, reproduction, and spread of *Bulinus* spp. snails analyzed.

Rate and transmission pattern of human infections

The investigation of *S. haematobium* infection was conducted among 100 adults (aged 20–55 years) and 100 primary school-aged children from first and second grades in every pilot area. Urine samples were collected every day from 10 am to 2 pm, and the infection was detected with the naked eye and then tested using the membrane filter method. Then, the infection rate and intensity of *S. haematobium* were calculated.

Consistently, 100 school-aged children (50 boys and 50 girls) and 100 adults (50 males and 50 females) are selected for baseline survey. All participants have undergone mass drug administration by praziquantel before the commencement of the pilot study. Then, the presence of *S. haematobium* is detected using the standard method, in the selected school-aged children and adults every two months from January to December. The infection rate and density of *S. haematobium* are calculated every two months to determine the transmission pattern of *S. haematobium* in Zanzibar.

Knowledge, attitudes, and practices (KAP) survey

One class from each grade in a primary school and 100 adults was randomly selected in the pilot area for an investigation on the KAP of schistosomiasis. Knowledge of schistosomiasis comprises its life history, diagnostic methods, main control measures, the compliance in chemotherapy, behavior types, and so on. The KAP survey was conducted by local health workers and Chinese experts.

Biological study of *Bulinus* spp. snails in laboratory

The *Bulinus* spp. snails captured in the field are bred in the laboratory which is located in Pemba, Zamziber. Schistosome egg production, egg hatching time, time from snail development to oviposition, duration of oviposition, and lifespan of *S. haemalobium* were tested under various temperatures. The reproduction rate, cumulative growth, and development temperatures of *S. haemalobium* were estimated to investigate the reproduction and growth pattern of snails.

Assessment of molluscicidal efficacy against *Bulinus* spp. snails in the laboratory and field

The efficacy of novel molluscicides developed in China against snails were assessed, while the WHO-prequalified 70% niclosamide ethanolamine salt wettable powder served as a control. The compounds are formulated into solutions with effective concentrations of 0.5, 0.25, 0.125, 0.063, 0.032, and 0.016 mg/L. Each solution was transferred to a 100-mL beaker. Then, 10 two-month-old snails were placed in each beaker covered with a stainless steel net to prevent the snails from escaping the solution. Following separate immersions for 24 and 48 hours, the solution were removed, and the snails were washed with dechlorinated water and bred in water for 48 hours. The mortality and median lethal concentration (LC_{50}) were estimated.

Based on the hydrographic survey and epidemiological investigation of snails, a small ditch or canal was divided into several segments in the study map, and the volume of the water body was measured. The amount of the molluscicide used was estimated according to the molluscicide dose. An immersion test was performed to evaluate the molluscicidal effect of two to three formulations of the molluscicides, each containing two to three doses. After immersion for one, three, and seven days, the snails were captured and stored in various containers. All snails were tested for LC_{50} in the laboratory, with the snail mortality or reduction of the snail density estimated. Following immersion for one or three months, the long-term molluscicidal effect was assessed. In each experiment, the air temperature and climate were recorded, with the study individual protected to prevent human and animal from infections through water contact.

5.4.6   The implementation of the intervention

The comprehensive intervention is put into effect in the pilot areas, according to the transmission patterns of *S. haematobium* and environmental features.

Treatment of humans adhere to preventive chemotherapy, taking place twice a year, as according to the National Plan of the Zanzibar Neglected Tropical Diseases Program. The coverage rate of chemotherapy must reach more than 90% (by the end of the project). Mollusciciding is conducted in all habitats of *Bulinus* spp. snails, which located in the pilot areas. Health education are carried out both for children and adutls, according to the early results in the KAP investigation.

5.4.7　Statistical analysis

Assessment indexes mainly include the infection rate and intensity of schistosomiasis in different groups of people, the distribution and density of *Bulinus* spp. snails, and the score of KAP pertaining to different groups of people.

Descriptive, correlation, and regression analyses; a cost-effectiveness/efficiency analysis; and a spatial analysis will be used to (i) analyze the epidemic and transmission pattern of schistosomiasis, thereby determining the feasibility of schistosomiasis control and elimination; (ii) screen comprehensive control measures in different levels of infection; (iii) analyze the cost-effectiveness/efficiency of the control measures; and (iv) access the control efficiency of comprehensive control measures through differential analysis.

In conclusion, Chinese experience in and expertise with schistosomiasis elimination, particularly with blocking its transmission, and the increasing needs in cooperation and collaboration with African countries, will prompt an integrated strategy that could be taken into effect in local setting of African countries. The success of such integrated studies would be an indicator to assess the feasibility in elimination of schistosomiasis in the African continent.

References

1.　Ross AG, Chau TN, Inobaya MT, et al. A new global strategy for the elimination of schistosomiasis. Int J Infect Dis, 2017; 54: 130-137.

2.　Lo NC, Addiss DG, Hotez PJ, et al. A call to strengthen the global strategy against schistosomiasis and soil-transmitted helminthiasis: the time is now. Lancet Infect Dis, 2017; 17: e64-e69.

3.　Wang X, Wang W, P. Wang. Long-term effectiveness of the integrated schistosomiasis control strategy with emphasis on infectious source control in China: a 10-year evaluation from 2005 to 2014. Parasitol Res, 2017; 116: 521-528.

4. Li YS, Zhao ZY, Ellis M, et al. Applications and outcomes of periodic epidemiological surveys for schistosomiasis and related economic evaluation in the People's Republic of China. Acta Trop, 2005; 96: 266-75.

5. Liu Y, Zhou YB, Li RZ, et al. Epidemiological features and effectiveness of schistosomiasis control programme in mountainous and hilly region of the People's Republic of China. Adv Parasitol, 2016; 92: 73-95.

6. Shi L, Li W, Wu F, et al. Epidemiological features and control progress of schistosomiasis in waterway-network region in the People's Republic of China. Adv Parasitol, 2016; 92: 97-116.

7. Xu J, Steinman P, Maybe D, et al.Evolution of the National Schistosomiasis Control Programmes in The People's Republic of China. Adv Parasitol, 2016; 92: 1-38.

8. Basch PF. Schistosomiasis in China: an update. Am J Chin Med, 1986; 14: 17-25.

9. Zhang W, Wong CM. Evaluation of the 1992-1999 World Bank Schistosomiasis Control Project in China. Acta Trop, 2003; 85: 303-13.

10. Song L, Wu X, Ning A, et al. Lessons from a 15-year-old boy with advanced schistosomiasis japonica in China: a case report. Parasitol Res, 2017; 116: 1787-1791.

11. Savioli L, Albonico M, Colley DG, et al. Building a global schistosomiasis alliance: an opportunity to join forces to fight inequality and rural poverty. Infect Dis Poverty, 2017; 6: 65.

12. Zoni AC, Catala L, Ault SK. Schistosomiasis prevalence and intensity of infection in Latin America and the Caribbean Countries, 1942-2014: A Systematic Review in the Context of a Regional Elimination Goal. PLoS Negl Trop Dis, 2016; 10: e0004493.

13. Zanzibar, http://zanzibar.go.tz.

14. Montresor A, Ramsan M, Chwaya HM, et al. School enrollment in Zanzibar linked to children's age and helminth infections. Trop Med Int Health, 2001; 6: 227-31.

15. Goatly KD, Jordan P. Schistosomiasis in Zanzibar and Pemba. East Afr Med J, 1965; 42: 1-9.

16. Knopp S, Person B, Ame SM, et al. Elimination of schistosomiasis transmission in Zanzibar: baseline findings before the onset of a randomized intervention trial. PLoS Negl Trop Dis, 2013; 7: e2474.

17. Stothard JR, French MD, IS Khamis, et al. The epidemiology and control of urinary schistosomiasis and soil-transmitted helminthiasis in schoolchildren on Unguja Island, Zanzibar. Trans R Soc Trop Med Hyg, 2009; 103: 1031-44.

18. French MD, Rollinson D, Basanez MG, et al. School-based control of urinary schistosomiasis

on Zanzibar, Tanzania: monitoring micro-haematuria with reagent strips as a rapid urological assessment. J Pediatr Urol, 2007; 3: 364-8.

19. Rollinson D, Klinger EV, Mgeni AF, et al. Urinary schistosomiasis on Zanzibar: application of two novel assays for the detection of excreted albumin and haemoglobin in urine. J Helminthol, 2005; 79: 199-206.

5.5 Case study: Global Fund malaria program in China, 2003–2013

5.5.1 Project title

China Global Fund malaria program

5.5.2 Founding and co-facilitating institutions

This project was financially supported by the Global Fund to HIV/AIDS, Tuberculosis, and Malaria (Global Fund). The project had been completed through co-cooptation of a large number of organizations, including the Country Coordinating Mechanism (CCM), Ministry of Health of China, the Chinese Centers for Disease Prevention and Control (CDCs), and non-governmental organizations (NGOs). The CCM for the Global Fund programs in China was established, which had the role of submitting funding applications to the Global Fund. Under the supervision of the CCM and the Ministry of Health of China, projects were implemented by CDCs at all levels, together with partners that included international NGOs.

The China CDC was appointed as the Principal Recipient (PR) and had the role of managing the China Global Fund programs. The PR consisted of nine departments, including the program office, financial department, procurement department, monitoring and evaluation (M&E) department, human resources department, audit department, as well as the National AIDS Program Office, National TB Program Office, and National Malaria Program Office (NMPO). The three national program offices were responsible for planning and implementing specific programs. Five rounds of malaria programming took place: Round 1 (R1), Round 5 (R5), Round 6 (R6), Round 10 (R10), and the National Strategy Application (NSA). The NMPOs of the China R1, R5, R6, and the NSA was located in the National Institute of Parasitic Diseases (NIPD), China CDC in Shanghai, while the R10 project was implemented in conjunction with the Yunnan Provincial Bureau of Health, according to the policy of MOH. The responsibility of the NMPO was to prepare the work plan, monitor and evaluate the process, submit annual reports, and financial and assets management. The PR issued a series of documents, such as program agreements, work plans, and the *Handbook of Management and Technology*, in conjunction with the launch of each round.

The CDCs at the provincial and county levels were appointed as subrecipients and sub-subrecipients, respectively, to conduct program-related activities, such as training, M&E, and finance management. Health departments at the provincial and county levels were responsible for supervising the programs. Township hospitals mainly carried out malaria diagnosis, treatment, and health education. Monitoring and evaluation activities, procurement activities, and financial and audit activities ensured that all programs were progressing smoothly.

Sixteen Global Fund programs were successfully applied for including five AIDS programs, six TB programs, and five malaria programs. Between 2002 and 2015, the Global Fund had disbursed an accumulative total of US$ 805 million in China (AIDS program: US$ 324 million, 40.3%; TB program: US$ 367 million, 45.5%; and malaria program, US$ 114 million, 14.2%).

5.5.3   Rationales

Since the establishment of the Global Fund in 2002, which was a new international health financial mechanism, three disease control processes have been promoted through partnerships between governments, civil societies, the private sector, and communities all over the world.

The China Global Fund malaria program is the largest, longest, and most extensive international cooperation project relating to malaria in China. The role of the program was to effectively promote the overall implementation of the NMCP (2006–2015) and the China Malaria Elimination Action Plan (2010–2020). By the end of 2012, reported indigenous malaria cases had dropped to below 10,000, the lowest number in malaria control history in China. Elements of the Global Fund project, such as the multistakeholder cooperation mechanism, have been rolled out nationally.

5.5.4　Project design

Goals of the five program rounds

From 2003 to 2013, five rounds of the program were successively conducted in China: R1, R5, R6, NSA, and R10 (Table 5.1). Rounds 1, 5, 6, and 10 supported malaria control activities to reduce malaria burden, and NSA mainly supported malaria elimination activities. Almost 578 million people were beneficiaries of these programs.

Implementation of the five rounds

The Global Fund program generally lasted for five years and was divided into two periods: Phase I (the first two years) and Phase II (the last three years). In 2011, the 25th Global Fund Board meeting decided that the following eligibility criteria for renewals applications would become effective starting in 2012: (i) Group of 20 (G20) upper-middle-income countries with less than an extreme disease burden will no longer be eligible for renewals of grants; and (ii) the counterpart financing and focus of proposal requirements under the policy on eligibility, counterpart financing and prioritization will apply. As a member country of the G20 upper-middle-income countries with less than an extreme malaria burden, it was decided that China would no longer be eligible for renewals of the program. Therefore, the NSA and R10 were concluded upon completion of the first phase of the program (Figure 5.6). Since 2014, the Global Fund has not supported malaria control and elimination in China.

The covering areas of the Global Fund malaria program gradually expanded from 47 counties in 10 provinces in 2003 to 762 counties in 20 provinces in 2010. The majority of the program areas were characterized by poverty and a high malaria burden.

R1

In 2002, Yunnan and Hainan Provinces in southern China were facing a serious malaria problem.[1] More than 70% of malaria patients in China came from these two provinces. Rapidly increasing migration in these areas resulted in a significant

Table 5.1   Goals of the China Global Fund malaria program, 2003–2013.

Round	Budget (US$)	Program area	Beneficiaries	Overall goal
R1 (Apr 2003 – Mar 2008)	6,347,448	47 counties in 10 provinces	9.3 million	Roll-back malaria in target provinces and control the spread of multidrug resistant malaria
R5 (Oct 2006 – Jun 2010)	31,161,319	121 counties in six provinces	63.8 million	Roll-back re-emerging malaria in central provinces and reduce the malaria burden in poor areas of central and southern China
R6 (Jul 2007 – Jun 2012)	11,865,704	12 counties in Yunnan province and four special regions of Myanmar	3.5 million	Reduce the malaria burden of Chinese migrant workers across the border in 12 counties in Yunnan, and reduce the malaria burden of local residents in four special regions of Myanmar that border Yunnan
NSA (Jul 2010 – Jun 2012)	63,436,279	762 counties in 20 provinces	500 million	Reduce indigenous malaria cases to zero in China (except in some border areas in Yunnan province) by 2015
R10 (Jan 2012 – Dec 2013)	5,080,078	Seven counties in Yunnan province and five special regions of Myanmar	Almost 2.2 million	Reduce the malaria burden in five special regions of Myanmar, monitor drug resistance against artemisinin and its derivatives, control the number of imported infections, and promote the elimination of malaria in China

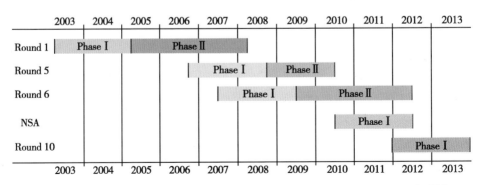

Figure 5.6   Road map of implementation of Global Fund malaria programs in China.

increase of malaria transmission. The risk of multidrug resistance spread in the border region of Yunnan and the mountainous areas of Hainan. Therefore, R1 was conducted to reduce the malaria burden and the risk of multidrug resistance in 25 border counties of Yunnan, 10 counties of Hainan, and 12 counties of another eight provinces (Henan, Hubei, Anhui, Jiangsu, Guangdong, Guangxi, Sichuan, and Guizhou). The main activities included: early diagnosis, appropriate treatment, and effective protection; malaria management among mobile populations in border areas of Yunnan; malaria-related health education and promotion; and malaria surveillance.

R5

Overall, 96% of the malaria cases in China in 2003 were reported from two southern provinces (Yunnan and Hainan), and four central provinces (Anhui, Hubei, Henan, and Jiangsu).[2] There was widespread antimalarial drug resistance in the high endemic areas of the southern provinces, and *Plasmodium vivax* malaria was rebounding in the central provinces. Round 5 was approved by the Global Fund to roll-back the reemergence of malaria in the central provinces and to reduce the burden of malaria in the southern provinces in 2005.

In the six provinces, 1,813 townships in 121 counties were selected as the target areas. This round pursued three strategic objectives: (i) malaria prevention; (ii) malaria diagnosis and treatment; and (iii) malaria surveillance and epidemic response. Malaria control capacity in the target areas was enhanced through the introduction of new techniques, including long lasting insecticidal nets (LLINs), rapid diagnostic tests (RDTs), and artemisinin-based combination therapies (ACTs), as well as multisectoral participation and health education.

R6

In China-Myanmar border areas, the burden of malaria was very high from 2001 to 2005. In Yunnan province, 25.6% of all malaria cases originated from the four special regions of northern Myanmar that border with China.[3] Among the Chinese migrants working cross-border, the risk of malaria was very high and difficult to reduce the malaria incidence in border areas. The surveillance and reporting systems for malaria were relatively weak in these special regions of Myanmar.

From 2006 to 2012, R6 was conducted to reduce the malaria burden of the border area, which included 12 counties in Yunnan and four special regions in northern Myanmar. The main goals of the R6 were to: (i) improve the malaria diagnosis and treatment for frequent migrant Chinese workers in Yunnan; (ii) improve the accessibility and quality of malaria prevention, diagnosis, and treatment for these migrant workers and local residents in the special regions; and (iii) determine the cross-border cooperation mechanism on malaria surveillance, information exchange, and joint control.

NSA

In 2008, the nationwide malaria situation in China met the pre-elimination criteria set out by the World Health Organization (WHO). The endemic areas were mostly poverty-stricken counties lacking the malaria elimination resources. To eliminate malaria in the entire country, the Global Fund approved the NSA proposal in 2009.

Unlike the previous stages that followed this "rounds" logic, the NSA was in line with China Malaria Elimination Action Plan, and included goals, objectives, indicators, and main activities. The NSA supported malaria elimination in endemic counties where local cases have been reported in three consecutive years. The target area of the NSA spread to the lower malaria burden provinces, whereas the previous grants only covered high malaria burden provinces. The government fund focused on other counties where there were no local cases reported in three consecutive years or non-malaria epidemic areas. With the principle of the one strategy plan and resource consolidation, the NSA consolidated two program grants (R5 and R6), and consolidated all the resources on malaria elimination in China. The objectives were to: (i) offer timely diagnosis and proper treatment to malaria patients, and improve malaria prevention; (ii) enhance malaria control of populations at high risk; and (iii) further improve the malaria surveillance system.

According to the original proposal, the NSA was intended to last five years. However, the program ended ahead of schedule on June 30, 2012, following the relevant decision of the Global Fund on G20 upper-middle-income countries with less than an extreme disease burden no longer are eligible for renewals of grants.

R10

The final China Global Fund malaria program round was R10. This round consolidated the achievments of malaria control in the China-Myanmar border area to continually reduce the malaria burden in the area and contribute to achieving malaria elimination in China.

Five special regions in Myanmar along the China-Myanmar border and seven border counties in Yunnan were selected as target areas. The target population included 586,000 local residents and 100,000 Chinese migrant workers in Myanmar, as well as 1.5 million frequent border crossers. The main activities were to: (i) improve accessibility of diagnosis and treatment; (ii) improve accessibility of LLINs; (iii) expand the coverage rate of preventive, diagnostic, and treatment services through information, education, and communication (IEC) and behavior change communication (BCC); and (iv) strengthen the efficiency of project management and information exchange.

5.5.5   Program input

Program fund

The Global Fund disbursed a total of US$ 114 million to support the Chinese malaria control and elimination programs, accounting for 14.2% of the total value of all Global Fund grants in China approved between 2003 and 2012. These funds played an important role in helping China to achieve its malaria control goals (Figure 5.7).

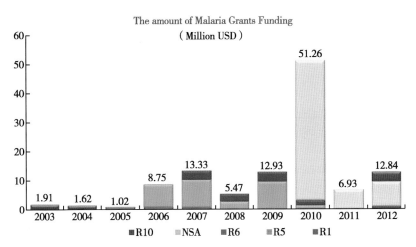

Figure 5.7   Annual amount and percentage by different rounds of Global Fund contributions to the Chinese malaria control program from 2003 to 2012.

Health products, equipment, and materials

From 2003 to 2012, the China Global Fund malaria program provided 5,516 micro-scopes; 6,655 sprayers; 967,560 RDTs; 2,399,069 person-doses of drugs; 1,823,153 LLINs; and 178,074 liters of pesticide for malaria diagnosis, treatment, and preven-tion. In addition, vehicles and office equipment improved the CDCs and facilitated program activities. These included 538 cars; 1,908 motorbikes; 1,461 computers; 1,012 cameras; 802 projectors; and 1,600 small fridges.

Human resources

The staff of CDC was responsible for most of the program activities, such as case test and treatment, vector control, malaria surveillance, and data management. The outlays of the CDC staff were provided by the governments at each level, but town-ship hospitals and village doctors were provided with incentives to improve case management and reporting. Due to human resource limitations, some partners (i.e. NGOs) recruited new staff to carry out malaria program activities.

For program staff, annual training in M&E, financial management, and pro-curement and supply was held at each level. The management capacity at each level was enhanced to ensure that the program was correctly implemented. (Re-) training courses on diagnosis, treatment, vector control, and surveillance were provided to a total of 444,941 trainees with support of the NSA. All township microscopists and 98.02% of the village doctors in program areas were (re-) trained. A sample survey of 27,499 township and village doctors in 2012 showed that 94.90% were satisfied with the training.

With the support of R5, about 15 persons gained their master's degree in public health management and technical specialties, some of which were related to the tech-nology or management of malaria control in China.

5.5.6 Program output

Over the 10-year duration of the program, about 1.40 million malaria cases (including suspected cases) were treated in a timely manner and 1.10 million patients infected in the previous year were treated, 2.80 million bed nets were treated with insecti-cides, and 1.80 million LLINs were distributed. A variety of local IEC/BCC materials were developed and distributed, and health education activities were carried out to improve the residents' awareness of malaria prevention and treatment.

Case management

For diagnosis, microscopy remained the gold standard throughout the program. The diagnostic options increased from only one method (microscopy) at the time of R1 to three methods (microscopy, RDTs, and polymerase chain reaction, PCR) during the NSA stage. From 2005 to 2010, 81 countries globally used RDTs for rapid malaria detection.[4] Rapid diagnostic tests were the primary diagnostic tool used in remote villages in southern China from 2008 to 2012. However, both microscopy and RDTs have lower sensitivities than PCR.[5] Polymerase chain reaction was mainly used for case verification in provincial CDCs and the NIPD, due to a lack of PCR equipment in county CDCs and townships.

The quality assurance (QA) system was updated by establishing a reference laboratories network, setting up microscopy oversight teams, and (re-) training microscopists. Microscopes and related materials were provided to township hospitals and malaria diagnoses were periodically double checked.

A total of 13 provincial reference laboratories were established, and all 762 counties in 20 provinces and autonomous regions set up microscopy monitoring groups for quality control. Rapid diagnostic tests were adopted to detect malaria in Yunnan, Hainan, Guizhou, and Tibet. A total of 12,485,598 fever patients received microscopic tests in the framework of R1, R6, and NSA.

Before 2010, case detection mainly relied on blood examination of fever patients in hospitals at all levels. Since the implementation of the NSA, in addition to blood examination, active case detection (ACD) was carried out to find infection sources.

Treatment competence was strengthened through special training and the provision of appropriate antimalarial drugs. In China, patients infected with *P. vivax* were treated with chloroquine/primaquine and patients infected with *P. falciparum* were treated with artemisinin therapy before R5. In 2006, ACTs for *P. falcipaum* and co-packaged chloroquine/primaquine for *P. vivax* were first used in program areas of R6. The National Malaria Treatment Policy was then revised to use ACTs as the first-line drug for treating *P. falciparum* infections, in line with international policy.

Artemisinin monotherapy for uncomplicated malaria was no longer to be used and injectable artesunate was used to treat severe or complicated malaria. In addition, *P. vivax* cases were treated with primaquine in periods of inactivity (usually in the Spring), which was named "Spring Treatment". The follow up for case treatment was provided by village doctors. Chinese Food and Drug Administration (CFDA) performed routine antimalarial drug quality control in the whole process, from production and circulation, to distribution and storage. A total of 1,504,613 confirmed and suspected malaria cases were treated between 2003 and 2012. Since 2004, each malaria case had been reported in a timely manner through the national infectious diseases reporting system network.

Vector control

Long lasting insecticide treated nets (LLINs) are a key malaria control strategy of relevant programs worldwide.[6] In highly endemic areas of Yunnan, Hainan, and Guizhou, LLINs were distributed and insecticide-treated nets (ITNs). Meanwhile, in four special regions of Myanmar, local residents and mobile populations also received LLINs through R6. Both the distribution of LLINs and ITNs were free of charge except in eight counties of Yunnan province, where LLINs were distributed through social marketing as an innovation model.

The distribution of LLINs were based on malaria incidence in program areas and the economic conditions of the households. Before 2010, all nets were treated once per year immediately before the malaria transmission season. The nets were treated with insecticide in the villages (incidence < 1% in the previous year) after 2010, and LLINs were provided only in a few villages (incidence ≥1% in the previous year). A total of 1.8 million LLINs were distributed and 3.56 million nets were treated with insecticide.

Net ownership can be significantly improved in a short time but net use is not always proportionally increased.[7] In 2012, 88.3% of at-risk households received at least one LLIN/ITN in the previous 12 months, and 65.1% of the at-risk population reported sleeping under a LLIN/ITN the previous night.

Indoor residual spraying was only used for vector control in confirmed transmission foci. In 2012, 3,941 foci received IRS and the effectiveness was assessed to ensure that residents received better malaria protection.

Health education and community mobilization

All provinces and partners carried out investigations on health education needs and developed locally appropriate information, education and communication/behaviour change commnication (IEC/BCC) methodologies and materials in conjunction with the various target groups. These included: 259,640 posters on malaria knowledge exhibited in public areas; 12,644 malaria health education courses held for primary and secondary school students; malaria programs broadcasted over radio or TV, 532 times in target counties; 276,617 families reached by face-to-face community activities; 133,455 primary/middle school students and 5,025 villagers trained on malaria knowledge; 2,079 village committees for malaria control established; 267,000 calendars and 7,000 posters delivered to mobile workers; 306.81 million pieces of IEC materials distribution or exhibited; health education activities conducted for 4,663 primary and middle school students in seven provinces; community health education activities conducted in 13 counties of Yunnan and 12 counties of Guizhou; 176,879 families visited by health workers in 3,115 villages of four counties in Yunnan; 100,000 people received health education; and 1.3 million IEC materials distributed at entry and exit ports. In Yunnan Province, for example, the printed materials consisted of local minority language calendars, notebooks, posters, videos, and so on. These were each targeted for different population needs of students, residents, and mobile cross-border workers.

A number of BCC activities were carried out by NGOs, the Chinese Ministry of Education (MoE), and CDCs by way of IEC material distribution, television and radio broadcasts, short messages systems (SMSs), websites, health education courses, community activities, face-to-face communication, and so on. About 400 million people received malaria health education. Since 2005, 26 April has been declared the "Chinese Malaria Day", immediately following World Malaria Day on 25 April. During Chinese Malaria Days, many IEC/BCC activities have been carried out all over the country (Figure 5.8).

Malaria control for populations at high risk

Pregnant women and children are the populations at high risk for malaria in Africa.

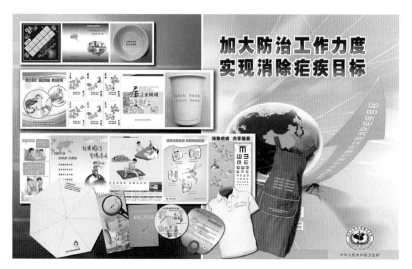

Figure 5.8   IEC, BCC materials designed by Global Fund malaira program.

However, the population at the highest risk for malaria in China is that exposed to risk factors related to work activities and location of residence. The population at the highest risk mainly includes the mobile population working across the border of Yunnan;[8] forest goers in Hainan; some ethnic minority peoples of Yunnan, Hainan, and Guizhou; and international migrants.

The key activities for populations at high risk were to expand coverage of malaria services such as LLINs, and IEC/BCC material distribution in coopera-tion with partners. Meanwhile, travelers from Africa and other endemic countries received IEC/BCC materials and RDT screening, which was also conducted at all ports. On the China-Myanmar border, eight mobile medical teams and 73 malaria consultation posts were established during R6 to provide malaria diagnosis and treatment services for mobile workers crossing the border. Malaria control activities among mobile workers involved in road construction or working on plantations and in forest areas were conducted in six program provinces during R5.

Malaria surveillance

The national malaria surveillance system was further improved, and the epidemic response capability at the county level was strengthened through training and the provision of equipment, RDTs, and insecticide for IRS. Surveillance technical skills trainings were held to improve the quality of case reporting.[9]

An antimalarial drug resistance surveillance network was set up during R5, R6, and the NSA stage, which included *in vivo* and *in vitro* monitoring of ACT and an *in vivo* study of chloroquine efficacy. Drug quality surveillance was termly carried out in Yunnan. Mosquitos density surveillance and insecticide resistance surveillance activities were carried out in 200 sentinel counties in the framework of the NSA. *In vitro* testing of sensitivity to antimalarial drugs was carried out along the China-Myanmar border with support of the Global Fund, as *P. falciparum* was found to have a high resistance to chloroquine in that area.[10] Artemisinin resistance in *P. falciparum* malaria was suspected in the China-Myanmar border area.[11]

Since 2010, every reported case has been followed up, resulting in 226,254 ACD activities involving 1,933,444 people.

Multisector cooperation

Throughout the program, multisector cooperation on malaria control and elimination was established and continued to be improved. Before 2003, no NGOs took part in malaria control in China, but with the launch of the Global Fund malaria program, some NGOs such as Health Unlimited/Health Poverty Action (HU/HPA) from the United Kingdom (UK), Humana People to People (HPP) from Zimbabwe, and Population Services International (PSI) from the United States (US) conducted many malaria control activities as partners. At first, they only took part in temporary activities such as monitoring and providing technical assistance during R1. Six partners conducted activities as subrecipients, including health education and promotion, LLIN distribution, antimalarial quality control, and malaria screening of the mobile population at border ports during R5. During R6, 70% of the funding was used for activities carried out by HU/HPA, and HPP. Especially, in the Myanmar border areas, malaria control was mainly carried out by HU/HPA. During the NSA, these partners continued to implement malaria elimination activities. Since R1, the WHO provided technical assistance to Chinese malaria control and elimination efforts and the China Global Fund malaria program. Meanwhile, especially in elimination areas, the private sector was engaged in malaria diagnosis, treatment, and reporting (Table 5.2).

Operational research

The NMPO developed application guide for operational research. Through public

Table 5.2 Partners of the Global Fund malaria program in China.

	HU/HPA	HPP	PSI	Red Cross Society of China (RCSC)	MoE	CFDA	China Entry-Exit Inspection and Quarantine (CIQ)	WHO
R1	M&E	–	–	M&E	–	–	–	Technical assistance
R5	Community health education	–	LLIN distribution through social marketing	LLIN distribution	Student health education	QA of antimalarials	Malaria screening at ports	Technical assistance
R6	Malaria control in Myanmar	Face-to-face health education	–	–	–	–	–	Technical assistance
NSA	Community health education	Face-to-face health education	–	LLIN distribution	Student health education	QA of antimalarials	Malaria screening at ports	Technical assistance
R10	Malaria control in Myanmar	–	–	–	–	–	Malaria screening at ports	Technical assistance

review, operational research proposals were selected and contracted. From 2007 to 2012, the program supported more than 40 operational researches that focused on the scientific problems of malaria control and elimination in China, primarily on topics such as genetic screening, vector control, malaria diagnosis, surveillance, imported malaria, treatment, and economic evaluation, etc. Some research results have been used to combat malaria and to provide technical support to malaria control and elimination activities.

5.5.7　Achievements and impact

In China, malaria incidence has decreased to below 1/10,000 at county level over the past 10 years. As the biggest international cooperation program focusing on malaria in China, the Global Fund was instrumental in this success.

Transition from malaria control to elimination

With the support of R1, the malaria burden in Yunnan and Hainan, the two provinces most severely affected by the disease, was significantly reduced. The number of malaria cases fell sharply from 6,357 to 1,844 in Hainan and from 13,816 to 4,027 in Yunnan between 2003 and 2008. With the support of R5, the prevalence of *P. falciparum* malaria shrunk to two provinces (Yunnan and Hainan). Under the joint promotion of the China Malaria Elimination Action Plan (2010–2020) and the NSA, malaria cases continued to decrease sharply from 7,855 in 2010 to 2,718 in 2012. The Chinese government and the Global Fund worked together to make malaria incidence (1/100,000) decrease from 3.91 in 2003 to 0.2 in 2012 (see Figure 2.4).

In 2011, the annual reported malaria incidence in 88.00% of the 75 high endemic counties was less than 1/10,000, and 21.33% of the 75 high endemic counties and 86.17% of the 687 middle and low endemic counties reported zero indigenous transmitted malaria cases

Over the 10-year period of the program, most notably in the framework of R1, R5, and the NSA, *P. falciparum* malaria was eliminated in Hainan. The incidence in the target counties of Hainan was 0.40/10,000 in 2007, and in 2011 there were no indigenous transmitted *P. falciparum* malaria cases. In Wanning City, which was previously a highly endemic area, transmission has dropped to zero since 2010.[12] In

Yunnan, *P. falciparum* malaria incidence dropped significantly year by year and was close to 0.118/10,000 in 2011.

From 2000 to 2006, malaria cases increased rapidly in four central provinces (Henan, Hubei, Jiangsu, and especially Anhui). The re-emergence of malaria was rolled back since R5 was launched in 2006. The incidence in only 10 counties in Anhui Province was still more than 1/1,000 in 2009. In Henan Province, the incidence of malaria decreased from 0.375/1,000 in 2006 to 0.047 /1,000 in 2010.[13] In Suining County of Jiangsu Province, malaria cases decreased from 37 cases to one case in the past five years, and the incidence decreased from 0.28/10,000 to 0.01/10,000, with a decline rate of 96.43%.[14]

In the China-Myanmar border area, R6 and R10 were implemented from 2007 to 2013. The malaria burden in four special regions of Myanmar was significantly reduced: the prevalence of malaria decreased by 94% among local residents in Myanmar.

Filling the resource gap for malaria control and elimination

Government funds for malaria control and elimination at different levels mainly covered human resources, logistics, overheads, and special fund for malaria control and elimination of non-project areas. The program areas were mostly poor and rural, with support focused on the weak links in malaria elimination such as diagnosis, treatment, monitoring, and awareness for malaria prevention. The existing funding gap was about 20% of the total malaria control and elimination budget in China, and was promptly filled by the Global Fund. Importantly, the Global Fund successfully leveraged the government at each level to increase funds for malaria control. For example, from 2003 to 2012, the central government invested about ¥ 193 million in malaria control and elimination, increasing from ¥ 5 million in 2003 to ¥ 46 million in 2012.

The health products and materials distributed by the Global Fund greatly eased the lack of resources for malaria control and elimination in China. Health products such as microscopes, insecticides, and RDTs filled the gap in malaria diagnosis and treatment in township hospitals, and LLINs boosted prevention of transmission. The procurement and distribution of materials such as vehicles and office equipment also provided necessary help for program implementation and malaria elimination.

Improved multisectoral cooperation and communication

Multisectoral cooperation and communication greatly benefited malaria control in China. Many government sectors and NGOs played important roles in malaria control. In the past, no NGOs had been engaged in malaria control in China. Besides the CDCs and NGOs (HU/HPA, HPP, and PSI), other government sectors, such as the MoE, CFDA, and the CIQ, as well as the Red Cross were involved in malaria control and elimination. Coordination meetings between CDCs and these partners were held regularly, and departments of tourism and commerce were also invited to attend these meetings. The number of provinces with multisectoral cooperation increased from six to 20 nationwide over the entirety of program duration. Together, these partners received 10% of the total funds from the Global Fund malaria program in China.

Contribution to policy-making and capacity-building in the NMCP

Malaria control and elimination policy in the fields of diagnosis, treatment, and vector control were revised over the course of program implementation. As new malaria control techniques such as RDTs, LLINs, and ACTs were introduced in China, these new techniques were integrated into the national malaria control policy and spread all over the country.

In terms of technical training, all microscopists, 98.02% of village doctors, and 63.41% of medical workers in township hospitals were (re-) trained. Nearly half of the microscopy staff working with grassroots organizations was trained several times. Thus, the program improved the comprehensive control and prevention abilities at all levels. The test scores related to blood slide preparation and readings were significantly higher in Global Fund-supported provinces than those not covered by the program.[15]

Program staff benefited from exposure to management concepts and improved their ability to manage programs, as well as the handling of M&E, procurement, financing, and audit.[16]

Enforcing public awareness of malaria control and prevention

Health education materials targeting different groups were developed and various health education activities were carried out to increase the malaria awareness rate.

More than 60% of the students among 44,519 students surveyed in 94 counties of 20 provinces in 2010 learned about the basic malaria knowledge.[17] In the four counties of Chongqing City, the percentage of primary school students who were aware of malaria increased from 58.94% to 89.96%, and the percentage of middle school students from 52.83% to 86.06%, and the percentage of local residents from 56.74% to 83.89%.[18] With the constantly improving awareness of malaria control and prevention, residents could go to hospital immediately if they became infected, and actively took part in malaria control and prevention activities.

Establishment of the cross-border cooperation mechanism for malaria control

The cross-border cooperation mechanism was established and enhanced during R6 and R10. Based on the platform of R6, the border counties in Yunnan and the special regions in Myanmar regularly exchanged and shared information on malaria. Technical assistance on malaria diagnosis and treatment was provided from Yunnan to the special regions in the form of human resources, training, and M&E. With the help of R6 and R10, the four special regions in Myanmar established a malaria network and system. Sixty-eight malaria control consultation and service posts in Yunnan and 73 health posts in Myanmar were established along the border. These health posts were equipped with microscopes and antimalarial drugs. The NGOs used 70% of the funds for malaria diagnosis and treatment, and health education in Myanmar. Meanwhile, there was strengthened mobilization and coordination between local health bureaus of special regions in Myanmar and those of the border counties in Yunnan, which improved the management and technical capacity of the officers from both countries.

References

1. Sheng HF, Zhou SS, Gu ZC, et al. Malaria situation in the People's Republic of China in 2002. Zhongguo Ji Sheng Chong Xue Yu Ji Sheng Chong Bing Za Zhi, 2003, 21: 193-196. (In Chinese)

2. Zhou SS, Tang LH, Sheng HF. Malaria situation in the People's Republic of China in 2003. Zhongguo Ji Sheng Chong Xue Yu Ji Sheng Chong Bing Za Zhi, 2005, 23: 385-387. (In Chinese)

3. Bi Y, Tong S. Poverty and malaria in the Yunnan province, China. Infect Dis Poverty, 2014, 3: 32.

4. Zhao JK, Lama M, Korenromp E, et al. Adoption of rapid diagnostic tests for the diagnosis

of malaria, a preliminary analysis of the Global Fund program data, 2005 to 2010. PLoS One, 2012, 7: e43549.

5. Yan J, Li N, Wei X, et al. Performance of two rapid diagnostic tests for malaria diagnosis at the China-Myanmar border area. Malar J, 2013, 12: 73.

6. Ghebreyesus TA, Lynch MC, Coll-Seck AW. The Global Malaria Action Plan for a Malaria-Free World. Roll Back Malaria Partnership, 2008.

7. Shargie EB, Ngondi J, Graves PM, et al. Rapid increase in ownership and use of long-lasting insecticidal nets and decrease in prevalence of malaria in three regional States of Ethiopia (2006-2007). J Trop Med. 2010; 2010. pii: 750978.

8. Chen GW, Wang J, Huang XZ, et al. Serological detection of malaria for people entering China from 19 ports of entry covering 8 border prefectures of Yunnan. Zhongguo Ji Sheng Chong Xue Yu Ji Sheng Chong Bing Za Zhi, 2010, 28: 54-57. (In Chinese)

9. Zhou XN, Bergquist R, Tanner M, et al. Elimination of tropical disease through surveillance and response. Infect Dis Poverty, 2013, 2: 1.

10. Zhang CL, Zhou HN, Wang J, et al. In vitro sensitivity of Plasmodium falciparum isolates from China-Myanmar border region to chloroquine, piperaquine and pyronaridine. Zhongguo Ji Sheng Chong Xue Yu Ji Sheng Chong Bing Za Zhi, 2012, 30: 41-44. (In Chinese)

11. Huang F, Tang LH, Yang HL, et al. Therapeutic efficacy of artesunate in the treatment of uncomplicated *Plasmodium falciparum* malaria and anti-malarial, drug-resistance marker polymorphisms in populations near the China-Myanmar border. Malar J, 2012, 11: 278.

12. Lin MH, Wen L, Wen SW, et al. Effect in implementation of Global Fund Malaria Project in previously high malaria-endemic area of Wanning City. Chin Trop Med, 2013, 13: 4. (In Chinese)

13. Liu Y, Guo XF, Zhang HW, et al. Evaluation of the Fifth Round of Projects Supported by the Global Fund to Fight HIV/AIDS, Tuberculosis, and Malaria in Henan Province. J Pathogen Biol, 2011, 6: 754-756. (In Chinese)

14. Tang YE. Effect of execution of Global Fund Malaria Project in Suining County. Zhongguo Xue Xi Chong Bing Fang Zhi Za Zhi, 2013, 25: 633-635. (In Chinese)

15. Fu Q, Li SZ, Wang Q, et al. Report of analysis of National Technique Competition for Diagnosis of Parasitic Diseases in 2011 II Analysis of capabilities of Plasmodium detection. Zhongguo Xue Xi Chong Bing Fang Zhi Za Zhi, 2012, 24: 274-278. (In Chinese)

16. Li L, Mao SL, Xiao, N, et al. Discussion on pattern of Global Fund Malaria Control Project in Sichuan Province. J Prev Med Inform, 2009, 25: 993-996. (In Chinese)

17. Yin JH, Wang RB, Xia ZG, et al. Students' awareness of malaria at the beginning of national malaria elimination programme in China. Malar J, 2013, 12: 237.

18. Wu CG, Luo F, Jiang SG, et al. Effect Evaluation of the awareness of knowledge about malaria: The Global Fund Malaria Project in Chongqing. Chin J Evid-based Med, 2013, 13: 1409-1412. (In Chinese)

5.6 Opportunities for international cooperation in parasitic disease control: China's foreign aid for public health

Foreign aid, also called international aid, overseas aid, or foreign assistance, is a voluntary transfer of resources from one country to another. The aid may be considered as a diplomatic approval to reward a government. The aid may be provided by private individuals, companies, non-government organizations (NGOs), or governments. Aid standard varies country by country. In contrast to aid, international cooperation is the process of groups of countries or organizations working or acting together for a common or mutual benefit.

Usually, foreign aid is a systematic national activity involving national foreign aid policy and global strategy, comprehensive national power and impact, and technical and logistical support. China has a long history of dedication to foreign aid to promote a friendly external environment, even when it was still poor. The following is a review of China's foreign aid, with a focus on public health.

5.6.1 History of China's foreign aid on public health

As soon as the People's Republic of China was established, the country launched its foreign aid program with a start from its neighboring countries like the North Korea and Vietnam.[1] In 1950, an initiative aid program took place to support the Democratic People's Republic of Korea and Vietnam. Since 1955, aid in a variety of forms has been extended to non-socialist developing countries. In 1956, China took its first aid action for the African continent. Among the variety of aid activities, aid for health has been outstanding. The first medical team was deployed to Algeria in 1963.[1] Since then, more than 20,000 person-times of Chinese medical teams have been dispatched in the form of one Chinese province assisting one African country. Currently, nearly 50 teams providing free medical services are still active in 48 countries of five continents.[1]

In November 2006, the former Chinese President, Hu Jintao, solemnly made commitments on the Forum on China-Africa Cooperation (FOCAC) to build 30 anti-malarial centers equipped with drugs and other equipment in Africa.[1] In December 2015, Chinese President Xi Jinping formally announced ten priority areas China-African cooperation plans with a budget of US$ 60 billion to support African development in all aspects. In short, cooperation between China and Africa has become even stronger, which results in mutual support and double wins in the long run.

5.6.2   Exploration of health foreign aid models

Health aid has played a very active role in China's foreign aid program. Many innovative models and mechanisms have been explored and set up, including bilateral and multilateral cooperation, among which the South-South cooperation has been regarded as a successful model, with its achievements been spoken highly of around the world.[2] In various contexts, human communication and exchange have further promoted the cooperation. In the new era, such a strong, friendly relationship has been expanded from foreign aid to a partnership, with an emphasis on equality and mutual respect.

Simultaneously, China has started and enlarged its public health support to other countries, even though medical aid is still a major approach. The cooperation on malaria control has been highlighted as one of the important aspects, contributing to human welfare and global malaria elimination as advocated by the World Health Assembly (WHA).[3] Below are examples that demonstrate the achievements.

China-Africa collaboration in malaria control

The China-Africa health cooperation, including collaboration on malaria control, has grown through the deployment of medical teams, the running of training programs, donation of medicines and medical equipment, and conducting joint research and academic exchanges. Due to strong competition with well-known international pharmaceutical groups, a few Chinese pharmaceutical enterprises are successfully undergoing pharmaceutical sale registration in dozens of African countries, which provides good opportunities for Chinese-produced medicines to be used in the African market. Donating antimalarial drugs, diagnostic kits, and relevant equipment; sending experts; and providing onsite trainings, have demonstrated the increasing commitment on the part of the Chinese government to support the malaria control and elimination program in Africa. An outstanding example is the Chinese government's aid in building antimalarial centers in 30 African countries and donating antimalarial drugs through a bilateral cooperation mechanism since 2006. The antimalarial centers have not only played an active role in the diagnosis and treatment of malaria cases, but also contributed to communication and capacity-building, including capacity improvement in local medical research. A successful field control example was in Comoros, where a pilot malaria elimination program has achieved a significant blocking of malaria transmission and a reduction in malaria cases with the support of China.[4]

China has also facilitated academic exchanges and training programs for African officials and technical personnel each year, especially in recent decades. Chinese institutions led by the National Institute of Parasitic Diseases (NIPD), Chinese Center for Disease Control and Prevention (China CDC) have organized a dozen training workshops and seminars on many topics, such as prevention and control of tropical diseases, malaria, schistosomiasis, and other neglected tropical diseases (NTDs) in developing counties. More than 300 technical staff and officials from more than 20 African countries have been trained with a focus on strategies and measures of malaria prevention and control in China. Most recently, more and more Chinese institutions have made efforts to strengthen their cooperation with various international agencies and foundations, such as the Bill & Melinda Gates Foundation, the World Health Organization (WHO), the Global Fund to Fight HIV/AIDS, Tuberculosis and Malaria (GFATM), Canadian International Development Research Centre, and the Department for International Development of the United Kingdom (UK-DIFD), under multilateral or bilateral cooperation mechanisms, which have provided many more opportunities to explore new ways in cooperation of malaria control and elimination.[5] Based on the experiences and the renewed interest inspired by the FOCAC, there are newly upcoming opportunities to further strengthen the

China-Africa cooperation in malaria control and elimination with the support of multilateral partnership mechanisms in collaboration with national and international agencies.

The innovative trilateral cooperation

Three initiations of an innovative trilateral cooperation on parasitic diseases have been carried out in the last five years. The first was the China-UK-Tanzania malaria project entitled "Application of an Integrated Strategy with Community-based Approaches and Strengthening the Health System to Control Malaria Effectively in Southern Tanzania", which was implemented in Tanzania and supported by UK-DFID and the Chinese government. The second was a trilateral cooperation between China, Australia, and Papua New Guinea (PNG), entitled "Australia-China-PNG Pilot Cooperation on Malaria Control", supported by both the Australian and Chinese governments. The third one was the China-WHO-Zanzibar Cooperation project on the control and elimination of schistosomiasis entitled "The China aid project of schistosomiasis control and elimination in Zanzibar", supported by the Chinese government and the WHO.

All the aforementioned trilateral cooperation projects have strengthened the cooperation on international development among the partners, which is quite different from the traditional mechanism of China's health aid with a focus on bilateral cooperation. In these three projects, a Memorandum of Understanding (MoU) of Development Cooperation Partnership was signed between the partners in order to further strengthen the existing cooperation among the partners.

China has supported programs on malaria or NTDs in other countries in some form for more than 30 years. China has prioritized malaria and schistosomiasis control in its South-South cooperation health assistance programs. It is also a key element of the policy platform of China's health engagement with African countries through the FOCAC. To date, China has not been a major health actor in the Pacific and its contributions have centered on deployment of medical teams. A medical team from Chongqing is currently working in the Port Moresby General Hospital of PNG. In late 2013, China announced that malaria control would become one of the prioritized areas for its growing aid support to the Asia-Pacific.

To ensure an efficient trilateral working mechanism, pilot cooperation is designed to take into account three jointly agreed principles. The aims of the cooperation is to: (i) support the local national malaria strategic plan, (ii) complement local national and international donors' initiatives, and (iii) use resources drawn from each of the three partners. The trilateral health cooperation (also called partnership) is a quite new collaboration mechanism and is very different from bilateral and other forms of cooperation. All activities planned in the project are conducted and progressed under joint efforts of the partners.

5.6.3　Opportunities and challenges of China's foreign aid for health

In the WHA held in May 2015, the Sustainable Development Goals (SDGs) and the Global Technical Strategy for Malaria 2016–2030 was approved and issued. Malaria, one of the three top priority public health problems, is no longer considered as a public threat in China, as the country has been implementing its malaria elimination action plan since 2010. However, as globalization acceleration, imported malaria cases have risen sharply due to mobile populations. Health cooperation in various forms and approaches through Chinese engagement will be very crucial in malaria control and elimination with the contribution of other countries. This will not only help prevent the re-introduction of the disease from other malaria endemic regions to China, but also contribute to the global malaria elimination process via shrinking of global endemic areas.[6]

Based on previously mentioned challenges and gaps, opportunities for scaling up Chinese involvement in malaria control and elimination in Africa may include the following: (i) funding for equipment and essential health infrastructure; (ii) extending the scope of Chinese medical teams; (iii) providing extensive training; (iv) implementing collaborative research (including on traditional medicines); (v) speeding up technical transfer for production of pharmaceutical products; (vi) strengthening health system functions including laboratory testing and case information reporting support; (vii) building surveillance and response systems, (viii) M&E; and (iv) health education.

To make an accelerated and sustainable impact on malaria control and elimination in Africa, the South–South cooperation on malaria should be aligned with cost-effective and evidence-based local strategic plans for malaria control and elimina-tion, with a focus on identifying needs, filling gaps, and leveraging all national, bilateral, and multilateral as well as private sector opportunities. Given that China has accumulated experience in implementing health policies and interventions, which could be shared with African and Pacific island countries, the Chinese contri-bution should be very significant. It should start with the Test, Treat, Track (T3) ini-tiative that was advocated by the WHO and all partners, and is also in great demand in endemic countries.[7] To align with the T3 approach, which focuses on scaling up diagnostic testing, treatment, and surveillance, T3 and the corresponding surveillance manuals were used in Namibia by the former WHO Director-General Dr. Margaret Chan in April 2012.[8] Each suspected case of malaria will be confirmed with a RDT, treated with an appropriate antimalarial medicine, and tracked by a local surveillance system. Joint country efforts could be made by scaling up access to malaria diagnos-tic testing, access to treatment at the community level with quality artemisinin-based antimalarial compound medicines, including lifesaving injectable artesunate, and strengthening the malaria surveillance system.

However, many challenges still remain that block the way towards global elimi-nation of malaria. There are several reasons why some highly endemic areas bear an overwhelming malaria burden. Most malaria infections are caused by *Plasmodium falciparum*, which causes a severe and fatal type of disease, and this is the case par-ticularly in the south Sahara in Africa.[9] These areas are home to the most efficient species of mosquitoes transmitting malaria. Moreover, poor infrastructure and sani-tation, and a lack of funding for vector control, diagnostic tests, and treatment are still challenges in many regions, especially in rural areas of African countries. Many countries also lack the infrastructure and resources necessary for sustained activities against malaria. As a result, very few benefited from historical efforts to eliminate malaria. In most highly endemic areas including Africa and Asia-Pacific, malaria is understood to be one of the biggest reasons causing poverty. The annual economic growth in countries with a high malaria transmission has been lower than in malaria-free countries. Malaria also has a direct and huge impact on human resources. Malaria not only results in the loss of life and productivity due to sickness and death, but also hampers children's schooling and socioeconomic development through both absenteeism and other damage related to severe malaria episodes such as lacking of labors. Additionally, the funding gap has affected the use and coverage of long lasting insecticidal nets (LLINs), and there is a risk of resurgence in several African countries. It is urgently needed to access diagnostics and treatment, which are influenced by certain factors.

At present, drug resistance has become a big concern. *Plasmodium falciparum-*resistance to chloroquine occurred in all of Africa last century, and there is widespread resistance to sulfadoxine-pyrimethamine as well. Ineffectiveness of *P. falciparum* to artemisinin-based combination therapies (ACTs), which was initiatively reported on the Thailand-Cambodia border, has since spread to more than five countries of the Greater Mekong Subregion, while ACTs are currently efficient in Africa and play a major lifesaving role in malaria treatment.[10] Almost all endemic countries in Africa have changed their policies to adopt ACTs for the treatment of all malaria cases including *P. falciparum*. Unfortunately, many African populations like using local traditional medicines, however, there is no systematic data about the safety and efficacy through clinical and pharmacological studies, or quality control data to support the formal registration and use of such medicines for the treatment and control of malaria. Moreover, most Sub-Saharan Africa countries are of significant concern due to their high levels of malaria transmission and reports of widespread insecticide resistance.

Recently, several international roundtable meeting and summits with a focus on Chinese health cooperation with endemic countries were held to explore more opportunities to strengthen an innovative partnership between China, Africa, and Asia-Pacific counties. These meetings brought leaders from China and these countries together to share information and experiences, to exchange progress and lessons learned, and to recommend how health cooperation could be strengthened and deepened through certain appropriate models or mechanisms. During these talks, the major challenges of malaria control and elimination in Africa and other disease endemic regions were identified. They are: (i) poor infrastructure, substandard health services, and control measures coverage; (ii) poor distribution and access to diagnostic services and availability of effective treatments; (iii) inadequate funding for vector control, diagnostic testing, treatment, and surveillance; (iv) weak cross-border malaria control; (v) slow response to drug and insecticide resistance threat; and (vi) the vicious cycle of poverty and malaria/NTDs.

To meet these challenges, the following six aspects have to be addressed:

- to get adequate domestic inputs and external funding for sustained commitment to malaria or schistosomiasis elimination;
- to enhance national disease control programs in the context of strengthening and developing a more efficient health system;
- to ensure free access to disease diagnosis and treatment for vulnerable populations such as children and pregnant women, in addition to universal access to LLINs;
- to build up human resource capacity at national, district, and community levels;
- to set up efficient logistics, information reporting, and surveillance systems;
- to establish an early warning and detection platform to respond to malaria epidemics and other potential public health threats.

In conclusion, China is willing and well prepared to support African and other disease endemic countries based on the principle of needs, willingness, and desire for participation in health. Among the aid activities, capacity-building of health human resources is one of the most important and sustainable supports. Meanwhile, the new relationship, called a partnership, has and will further lead to achievements of mutual learning and double wins.

References

1. Global Health Research Center of Beijing University. China-Africa Health Collaboration in the Era of Global Health Diplomacy. Beijing: the World Knowledge Press, 2012.

2. Global Health Research Center of Beijing University. The Pathfinder in New Phase of China-Africa Health Cooperation. Beijing: the World Knowledge Press, 2013.

3. World Health Organization. Health in 2015 from MDGs to SDGs. WHO, 2015.

4. Deng C, Huang B, Wang Q, et al. Large-scale Artemisinin-Piperaquine Mass Drug Administration With or Without Primaquine Dramatically Reduces Malaria in a Highly Endemic Region of Africa. Clin Infect Dis, 2018; 67: 1670-76.

5. Ernest T, Ugwu CE, Guan YY, et al. China-Africa Health Development Initiatives: Benefits and Implications for Shaping Innovative and Evidence-informed National Health Policies and

Programs in Sub-saharan African Countries. Inter J MCH AIDS, 2016, (5): 119-133.

6. Li ZJ, Yang YC, Xiao N, et al. Malaria Imported from Ghana by Returning Gold Miners, China, 2013. Emerging Infect Dis, 2015, 21(5): 864-867.

7. World Health Organization. Scaling up diagnostic testing treatment and surveillance for malaria. WHO, 2012.

8. Smith JL, Auala J, Tambo M, et al. Spatial clustering of patent and sub-patent malaria infections in northern Namibia: Implications for surveillance and response strategies for elimination. PLoS One, 2017, 12(8): e0180845.

9. World Health Organization. World Malaria Report 2017. WHO, 2018.

10. World Health Organization. Approaches for mobile and migrant populations in the context of malaria multi-drug resistance and malaria elimination in the Greater Mekong Subregion. WHO, 2016.

图书在版编目（CIP）数据

中国公共卫生：热带病防治实践. 被忽视热带病与
疟疾 = Tropical Diseases in China：Neglected
Tropical Diseases and Malaria：英文 / 周晓农主编
. —北京：人民卫生出版社，2019
ISBN 978-7-117-28427-1

Ⅰ. ①中… Ⅱ. ①周… Ⅲ. ①热带病－防治－中国－
英文②疟疾－防治－中国－英文 Ⅳ. ①R599.3
②R531.3

中国版本图书馆 CIP 数据核字（2019）第 072227 号

人卫智网	**www.ipmph.com**	医学教育、学术、考试、健康， 购书智慧智能综合服务平台
人卫官网	**www.pmph.com**	人卫官方资讯发布平台

中国公共卫生：热带病防治实践. 被忽视热带病与疟疾（英文版）

主　　编：周晓农
出版发行：人民卫生出版社（中继线 010-59780011）
地　　址：北京市朝阳区潘家园南里 19 号
邮　　编：100021
E － mail：pmph @ pmph.com
购书热线：010-59787592　010-59787584　010-65264830
印　　刷：北京盛通印刷股份有限公司
经　　销：新华书店
开　　本：710 × 1000　1/16　印张：17.5
字　　数：305 千字
版　　次：2019 年 7 月第 1 版　2019 年 7 月第 1 版第 1 次印刷
标准书号：ISBN 978-7-117-28427-1
打击盗版举报电话：**010-59787491**　**E-mail：WQ @ pmph.com**
（凡属印装质量问题请与本社市场营销中心联系退换）